Collapse
and Resiliency

Collapse and Resiliency

The Inside Story
of Liberia's Unprecedented
Ebola Response

TOLBERT NYENSWAH, LLB, MPH, DrPH
With Mardia Stone, MD, MPH

FOREWORD BY
Former Liberian President
Ellen Johnson Sirleaf

JOHNS HOPKINS UNIVERSITY PRESS | *Baltimore*

© 2023 Tolbert Nyenswah and Mardia Stone
All rights reserved. Published 2023
Printed in the United States of America on acid-free paper
9 8 7 6 5 4 3 2 1

Johns Hopkins University Press
2715 North Charles Street
Baltimore, Maryland 21218
www.press.jhu.edu

Library of Congress Cataloging-in-Publication Data is available.

ISBN 978-1-4214-4755-1 (paperback)
ISBN 978-1-4214-4756-8 (ebook)

A catalog record for this book is available from the British Library.

All photos are by Mardia Stone unless otherwise noted.

Special discounts are available for bulk purchases of this book. For more information, please contact Special Sales at specialsales@jh.edu.

In memory of my beloved father, Moses, and to my loving mother, Ruth, for their endless love, support, and sacrifices. You are the greatest factors contributing to my lifetime of achievements.

AND

In loving memory of all health care workers and the thousands of Liberians who lost their lives to the deadly Ebola virus disease epidemic in Liberia.

CONTENTS

Foreword, by Ellen Johnson Sirleaf   ix
Preface   xix

Introduction   1

1. Ebola Hits Liberia   5

2. Born for Such a Time   20

3. Unsafe Rituals, Burial Practices, and International Spread   37

4. A Refugee in Côte d'Ivoire   49

5. Total Collapse of Public Health Care Services   75

6. Security Challenge: Community Distrust and Resistance—
   West Point   92

7. Interventions: What We Did and How We Did It   111
   Contact Tracing | Case Management | Epidemiology and Surveillance | Community
   Engagement and Social Mobilization | Laboratory Testing | Psychosocial
   Support | Dead Body Management | Logistics and Support Services | Finance and
   Administration | Health Care Workers | Airport, Seaport, and Land Borders

8. The International Response   139
   World Health Organization | African Union | United States | Médecins Sans
   Frontières (Belgium) | UNMEER | UNICEF | European Union | People's Republic
   of China | Cuba | Germany | World Bank | World Food Programme | Media |
   Nongovernmental Organizations

9. Recovery, Rebuilding, and Resiliency   177

10. Reflections   193

Acronyms and Abbreviations   209
References   213
Index   229

When one has been moved to laughter and tears—as well as ushered into modes of deep contemplation and insight—as I was while reading *Collapse and Resiliency: The Inside Story of Liberia's Unprecedented Ebola Response*, it is difficult to find a word or phrase to describe such an enriching experience. I find this book deeply inspiring.

This is a story of a man who emerged from humble beginnings in a rural village to become a hero in Liberia, a man who was instrumental in containing the deadly Ebola virus outbreak that ravaged our nation. The book is narrated in ten chapters. In the first chapter, Tolbert Nyenswah recounts the proliferation of tragedy that began in March 2014, when Liberia was plagued by the Ebola virus outbreak, which became the largest disease epidemic in recent global public health history. The outbreak started in Guinea and moved to Liberia and Sierra Leone, with over 28,000 people infected cumulatively. Of this number, 11,000 died before May 2016, when the outbreak was declared over by the World Health Organization. Liberia became the epicenter of this scourge. There were more than 11,000 cases and 4,800 deaths in our country alone. During that horrible two-year period, we faced the dread of an unknown enemy that indiscriminately claimed the lives of thousands of our citizens. It was a disaster of unimaginable proportions.

In chapter 2, "Born for Such a Time," Nyenswah documents his life story from childhood to adulthood, detailing later in chapter 4, "A Refugee in Côte d'Ivoire," the horrendous experiences he endured as a refugee fleeing his homeland to Côte d'Ivoire during the protracted Liberian civil war. He tells the story of unwavering parental guidance and support, courage, and perseverance throughout his life, becoming the leader his father had dreamed he would become from the day he was born. These experiences readied him for the principal role he would assume at a critical period in our nation's history.

Unsafe rituals, burial practices, and international spread are discussed in chapter 3, highlighting the conflicts between traditional practices and public health. Despite visible anti-Ebola messages disseminated all over the country and through nationwide radio broadcasts, members of traditional societies—rural and urban—continued to engage in unsafe rituals and burial practices. They touched, bathed, and dressed the dead, and exposed their children to infected corpses. Some even had secret burials without reporting the deaths to health authorities. Consequently, whole households and families became infected and died following these clandestine funerals. Convincing people to forgo such practices was a difficult task.

As infected Ebola corpses were thrown out of homes onto the streets of the capital city, Monrovia, the risk of transmission to local communities increased drastically. To address this issue, a Dead Body Management team was established to safely remove corpses from the streets and from people's homes to safely bury them. The situation prompted the government to consider cremation—a concept foreign to Liberian culture. People were fearful, believing that they would suffer damnation if cremated. For this reason, people stopped taking sick relatives to the treatment centers while continuing to handle, prepare, and secretly bury their dead. In August 2014, I mandated that all Ebola corpses be cremated, to discourage families from dumping dead relatives into the streets and to prevent transmission from highly contagious corpses.

Nyenswah writes of Patrick Sawyer, a naturalized Liberian-American citizen who traveled to Lagos from Liberia in July 2014. After Sawyer was diagnosed with Ebola at a local hospital and died, alarm grew of the possibility of international transmission and the likelihood of the disease spreading both regionally and across the Atlantic. The epidemic suddenly became a regional public health emergency. He also writes about Dr. Kent Brantley and Nancy Writebol, two American missionaries who also became infected in July while working in Liberia and were evacuated by private air ambulance to the United States. Brother Miguel Pajares, a Spanish volunteer infected in Liberia in early August, was evacuated to Spain by the Spanish military. Yet infected Liberians working for the same institutions received no such preferential treatment or consideration, creating public outcry and more demands on the government. On August 6, as cases began to escalate in the nation, I declared on national television a state of emergency and imposed a nationwide dusk-to-dawn curfew.

Our health system was devastated. In chapter 5, "Total Collapse of Public Health Care Services," Nyenswah addresses the decline in routine health services over a five-month period (August to December 2014). Health facilities (public and private) closed, health care workers refused to go to work for fear of their own health, and people chose not to seek care, even at facilities that remained opened. They distrusted the safety of these facilities or were refused care because the staff themselves were afraid of contracting Ebola. Pregnant women in labor suffered this fate all over the country, as they were refused admission by staff, fearing exposure to their blood.

Security concerns and issues relating to community resistance are presented in chapter 6, "Security Challenge: Community Distrust and Resistance—West Point." This chapter focuses on West Point, a densely populated beach slum on the outskirts of Monrovia, which became the site of the Ebola virus disease onslaught in early August. The Ministry of Health and Social Welfare set up a temporary isolation unit, in and specifically for the West Point community, to remove sick people from their homes and off the streets. When word got out, sick folks from other communities around Monrovia descended on the West Point isolation center, in desperate search of care and treatment. This infuriated West Point residents, who felt the center was theirs only. Looting of the isolation center and rioting ensued, prompting the government to respond by instituting firm public health and security measures, imposing a strict quarantine of the entire West Point area. The military and police were sent to enforce these measures and stop the riot. Angered by the deployment of the military—armed soldiers and police—in their community, crowds of residents clashed with police.

When I was informed of the situation, I immediately convened a meeting with my cabinet. We agreed that the quarantine on West Point be elevated and a dusk-to-dawn curfew be strictly enforced. Upon the recommendation of security forces, and acting on presidential directives, more riot police and soldiers moved into West Point with tanks, scrap wood, and barbed wire to seal off the area. We had to halt the epidemic; we believed then, that in this way, we could control Ebola transmission. There was gunfire, a young boy was killed, and several others were seriously injured. This heightened community anger and intensified their resistance. They no longer trusted the government, loudly vocalizing their discontent, and the quarantine turned into a volatile situation.

On August 19, I addressed the nation in a radio broadcast saying: "We have been unable to control the spread of Ebola due to continued denials, cultural burying practices, disregard for the advice of health workers, and disrespect for the warnings by the government. . . . Fellow citizens, these measures are meant to save lives." The following day, in addition to the existing quarantine isolating West Point, I extended the local curfew into a nationwide curfew, from 6 p.m. to 6 a.m., and dispatched the Liberian National Coast Guard to patrol the surrounding waters of West Point. Certainly, a less invasive approach would have been advisable or preferred to gain community acceptance. Perhaps, had we employed a community-based approach, engaged community leaders, and addressed their concerns and constraints we would have better prepared the community for the intervention. As such, military force would not have been necessary. On August 30, we ended the quarantine, giving the people of West Point some relief. However, for the wider population, the end of Ebola was not on the horizon.

On August 6, 2014, I declared a national state of emergency, the goal being to halt Ebola transmission and appropriately care for the afflicted. The World Health Organization also recognized the West African

Ebola epidemic as a global public health crisis. For our nation, it was critical that our actions were decisive, to better coordinate response activities nationwide, while tracking and managing the inflow of aid from various external donors.

On August 11, 2014, at the height of the Ebola epidemic, I appointed Tolbert Nyenswah as incident manager to lead the national Ebola response in Liberia. He demonstrated the utmost leadership capabilities, putting his life and the lives of his family members on the line when he accepted and committed himself to spearheading the incident management system (IMS) without hesitation. I became aware of this young man at one of our meetings in which we were discussing what the best coordination mechanism would be for an effective response. In methodical detail, Nyenswah presented the IMS concept and explained how it would operate. Although he was a junior minister at the time, I was impressed with the manner in which he made a case for adopting a system senior officials were unconvinced would be the best course. Articulating his reasons clearly and fearlessly, he was persistent in spite of contrary views voiced by his superiors. Given the scale of the epidemic and having tremendous confidence in his ability as a manager, I knew then that I had made the right decision in choosing him to lead our country out of a catastrophe. He was already prepared to shoulder his duty as incident manager.

Collapse and Resiliency gives you an understanding of Liberia's Ebola outbreak response, what we did to overcome the epidemic, and how it was accomplished, as detailed in chapter 7. The book presents the workings of the incident management system as the coordination mechanism for the response, describing the interventions we employed, and the way in which they were implemented. Nyenswah documents support from domestic and international sources, with the Ministry of Health and Social Welfare at the helm. This section identifies several thematic areas: Case Management (case isolation, screening of travelers, restriction of movement, and border control); Contact Tracing (active case search, active case finding, and contact listing); Epidemiologic Surveillance (tracking disease trends and control); Laboratory (sample collection and attendant safety methods, transport, testing, and reporting); Safe and Dignified Burials (collection of corpses from homes and other locations, training burial teams across the country, culturally sensitive burials, cremation, and citizens' resistance); Social Mobilization and Community Engagement (mobilizing and engaging the community in raising awareness about Ebola, involving faith leaders in the process, and addressing harmful traditions and practices that facilitated the spread of the disease); Psychosocial Support (dealing with the sick and dying, families affected by death of loved ones while mourning their loss, mental and psychological states of survivors who were infected and recovered, and regarding Ebola survivors with compassion); and International Response (participation of the African Union, Economic Community of West African States, United Nations agencies, the United States government, other foreign governments [including China and Cuba], aid agencies, and participation of nongovernmental organizations).

In chapter 8, "The International Response," this book notes the organizations that came to aid the nation and the roles they played in this seemingly relentless struggle. The World Health Organization was a key player and our lead technical partner in health. Together with the Ministry of Health, they initially led the response by providing guidance, technical expertise, and support for the direction the response would take. Médecins Sans Frontières / Doctors Without Borders set up the second and largest Ebola treatment unit in Monrovia. The African Union pooled together funding, human resources, and technical expertise from the Economic Community of West African States under the umbrella of the African Union Support to Ebola in West Africa, in support of West African subregional efforts, by dispatching African medics, epidemiologists, laboratory specialists, and other public health experts to tackle the Ebola crisis in the three affected member states. These efforts paid off, because together we conquered Ebola, thereby averting overwhelming subregional transmission of this deadly disease. The government of the People's Republic of China was the first to respond, sending a planeload of much-needed medical supplies and equipment, as well as medics and military personnel who set up an Ebola treatment unit. The European Union provided support, through technical experts, and other personnel from member states. A number of United States governmental agencies, including the US Embassy in Liberia, Centers for Disease Control and Prevention, the US Agency for International Development, and the Department of Defense, provided technical expertise and support, logistics, and military personnel to build Ebola treatment units. Local and international nongovernmental organizations, such as the Liberian Red Cross and the International Federation of Red Cross and Red Crescents, handled the management of corpses in addition to safe and dignified burials. The United Nations, through its various agencies, provided guidance, funding, relevant technical support, and logistics. The World Bank was a major funding source for most of what we accomplished during the response.

Chapter 9, "Recovery, Rebuilding, and Resiliency," discusses the restoration of routine health services that provide care and treatment to those with acute and chronic illnesses unrelated to Ebola. Contact tracing was enhanced as the system became better organized and simplified; rapid isolation and treatment of Ebola (RITE) patients was more organized and made easier with an increase in the number of treatment units in the country; community engagement, keeping the community involved and aware of developments and changes in the response as they occurred; coordination, logistics, and finance were important for an effective and consistent response. The incident management system grew stronger and coordination was more structured; logistics required pooling together resources from various sources and making them available for county incident management systems to operate more easily and fully; resurgence of cases, when they occurred, were handled more rapidly, isolation and testing more immediate, and case management more controlled. We considered not only recovery but future preparation, aimed at building a resilient health system in order to prevent, detect, respond to, and control any infectious disease, up to the magnitude of Ebola, that threatens the public health of our country. With this in mind, the Ministry of Health devised a scheme, crafting the Investment Plan for Building a Resilient Health System. This plan has nine pillars, the third pillar of which emphasizes building a strong public health infrastructure that would prevent any future threats. We also sought to establish Liberia's own public health institute, which would conduct nationwide epidemiologic surveillance toward disease prevention, maintain preparedness in threat detection, and map out the ability to respond effectively in averting disease outbreaks on the scale of Ebola. The National Public Health Institute of Liberia was conceptualized and, through many processes, a legislative act to establish the institute, which I signed, was passed into law on December 27, 2016. The National Public Health Institute of Liberia was officially established on January 26, 2017, and is now in full operation.

In "Reflections," chapter 10, Tolbert Nyenswah looks back and considers Liberia's Ebola response as "one of the most rewarding and demanding experiences of our lives . . . a pivotal moment"—a dream manifested. He reflects on what led to its success: behavioral change, the command-and-control incident management system, the government regarding the Ebola virus disease as a threat to the nation's "economic, political and social fabric," and the political leadership, which could not be substituted; a supporting cast of committed Liberian professionals, response structures that were established early on, and the government owning its response; navigating delicately the array of foreign partnerships in a multinational and multidisciplinary response, and emphasizing our slogan *One Plan, One Strategy, One Response*, by constantly reminding our partners and friends alike that the government was in charge; integrating national and foreign teams to work as specified thematic units made us recognize that foreign experts didn't know any more about managing Ebola than we did, which motivated us to be fully committed to being more self-reliant.

Nyenswah opines that Ebola may have been "a blessing in disguise" and, even though future epidemics or pandemics may emerge, the West African Ebola epidemic has already impacted the future of global public health. We reflect on African scientists who came to Liberia, having more knowledge, experience, and skills than their non-African counterparts, yet had worked in the shadows of others until then. Dr. Jean-Jacques Muyembe is a case in point. He first discovered Ebola in Congo (previously Zaire) in 1976, yet he was never recognized or credited by the Belgians to whom he sent samples for analysis. We acknowledge and applaud our fellow African scientists with gratitude for helping us save Liberia from annihilation by Ebola. We are also appreciative of all foreign entities that came to assist us.

Despite our national trauma experienced during the epidemic, Liberians continued to live their lives, even with the restrictions on common human interactions. Yet there was hope. The Monrovia Marathon, held on November 8, 2015, was, as its theme depicted, "A New Beginning"—people saw a reason to participate and celebrate life. It was the first regional, multinational sporting event post-Ebola. People crossed over from Sierra Leone and Guinea, with whom we shared the classification of "the three most affected countries" in the West African Ebola outbreak. Participants came from Kenya, Senegal, and other countries. Some had run in marathons in other parts of the world. It was truly a "new beginning," a fresh start, standing up against Ebola, and we prevailed.

By November 2014 we saw a significant drop from approximately one hundred new cases per day at the peak of the epidemic to ten confirmed new cases per day. Our six active laboratories tested sixty samples a day but on average only discovered eight new Ebola cases per day. Over a thousand people—including more than three hundred children, many of them orphaned—survived Ebola, recovered, and walked away free from disease. Liberians took our country's destiny into their own hands and replaced hopelessness with optimism. They understood their fears and therefore became more relieved. Nyenswah became a household name in Liberia, known as a true public servant, a man of strong character, a great strategist, and a national hero. As US General Norman Schwarzkopf said, "Leadership is a potent combination of strategy and character. But if you must be without one, be without the strategy."

I can confidently say that Tolbert Nyenswah is endowed as a highly skilled leader, recognized around the world. And, as proven, he had a masterful approach in place to beat Ebola out of Liberia.

Collapse and Resiliency will inspire you to believe that dreams do come true despite the odds. It will show you that family is important. It will show you that parental guidance, nurturing, and unwavering support will give you the strength to persevere when undue hardship overwhelms you. It will show you that with dedication, belief in yourself, and a determined spirit, dreams do become a reality. This is a book that will alter your thinking and give you a clear understanding of what leadership looks like in times of crisis.

Ellen Johnson Sirleaf
FORMER PRESIDENT, REPUBLIC OF LIBERIA

The idea to write this book originated from a discussion I had with my senior and technical advisor, Dr. Mardia Stone, at the end of the epidemic, when we were in the planning stages of creating the National Public Health Institute of Liberia. She conceived the idea that we write a book about the Ebola experience and tell the story, emphasizing the role I played. At the time, there had been so many articles, presentations, and even pending books or publications written by expatriates who claimed expertise or presumed to know everything about what we did in our response, without consulting me or other members of our team or even giving us credit (and often without even mentioning the names of those of us who managed Liberia's Ebola response). Dr. Stone was insistent that we had to write this book because no one else could tell the story better than the one who actually led the response.

And so, we began the process of in-depth discussions, interviews with me, discussions with my wife and other members of my family, to get their perspective of the role they played in supporting me as incident manager during the height of the epidemic, addressing their concerns and their fears. Meanwhile, as we drafted the first manuscript, numerous foreign nationals began to approach me about writing "The Ebola book." I declined their offers because I knew undoubtedly that the story I had to tell could best be told by me and not by anyone—particularly, not by anyone without the cultural and national perspective that I have. We submitted a proposal to Johns Hopkins University Press, my alma mater, which was accepted. And here we are, with the finished product—a book I believe you will find engaging.

I strongly believe that this book is important because it is written from my personal perspective as the man who led Liberia out of Ebola's pit of doom to freedom from the dreaded disease. I am one of the few people in the world who is truly qualified to tell this story. The events that occurred in Liberia with regard to how the Ebola outbreak was handled are important from an historic perspective, from lessons we learned on how to prevent and even more importantly, what to do in the event of future Ebola or other infectious disease outbreaks in Liberia or elsewhere in the world. I believe this will be an important text for students and the interested public. We address the challenges, uncertainties, conflicts, and missteps we encountered during the Ebola response. We address the interpersonal rivalries and differing agendas between various international organizations. We also address the issue of extravagance and waste and Ebola being a cash cow, even for organizations that did not previously exist until Ebola. Yet despite all the problems and apparent limitations, we were successful in curbing the epidemic. What we did and how we did it, what we would do differently, and the recommendations we would make to others are all presented in the ten chapters of this book.

ACKNOWLEDGMENTS

During my life, God has blessed me by exposing me to extraordinary people who have provided a strong network of support. I express my deep sense of gratitude and indebtedness to my beloved parents, William K. Moses Nyenswah (1932–2008) and Ruth Tanneh Moses Nyenswah, for nurturing, loving, and carrying me in every way possible. They gave me the strength to reach for the stars and follow my dreams. I am eternally grateful for my mother's unending prayers every moment I stepped out to manage the Ebola response.

I am particularly honored to acknowledge the former president of the Republic of Liberia Ellen Johnson Sirleaf for recognizing me as a leader and bestowing upon me such Herculean responsibility.

My warmest thanks to my darling wife, Josephine Kikeh Nyenswah, for her unconditional love, devotion, support, and unwavering belief in me. She has inspired me in all dimensions of my life. I thank my children, Dehkontee, Nyennekon, and Tolbert Jr., for being understanding and supportive during the darkest days of the outbreak when they were afraid that I would come home infected with Ebola. They were also very cooperative during the period while we were writing this book, that they made all efforts to keep stress away from me. You share the credit for every goal I achieve.

I would like to acknowledge the following groups and individuals:

Government of the Republic of Liberia: Thanks to Hon. Augustine K. Ngafuan, former minister of foreign affairs, and former minister of finance and development planning, who, with the help of President Sirleaf, mobilized our foreign partners. He also personally hand carried the small shipment of ZMapp drug to Liberia when it was granted to the government for compassionate use. Dr. Walter T. Gwenigale, former minister of health and social welfare (posthumously); Dr. Bernice T. Dahn, former minister of health, deputy minister of health, and chief medical officer (CMO), for believing in me, when she made me her assistant minister, deputy CMO and for her confidence in my ability to spearhead the incident management system; Hon. Amara Konneh, former minister of finance and development planning, for standing by me and supporting me, even though I was a junior minister, and for encouraging other cabinet ministers to do the same; Hon. Morris Dukuly, former minister of internal affairs; Hon. Brownie Samukai, former minister of national defense, who mobilized the military and supported the civil authority; Hon. Lewis Brown, former minister of information, cultural affairs, and tourism, for creating a platform for synchronized communication and information dissemination to the public; Mrs. Jessie E. Duncan, former assistant minister of health for preventive services and deputy chief medical officer; Ms. Mary Broh, director general, General Services Agency; Mr. Dehpue Zuo, former deputy minister, international cooperation, Ministry of Foreign Affairs; the Senate and House of Representatives 53rd Legislature, with special mention to Hon. Edwin Melvin Snowe for his support and encouragement; Hon. Saah H. Joseph, former representative; Dr. Peter S. Coleman, former senator and chair of the Senate Committee on Health for his continuous advice and presence on the IMS; the Judiciary; the Armed Forces of Liberia; and local government officials who stood towering during the call to action throughout the outbreak.

Republic of Liberia's incident management system team: Dr. Emmanual Dolo (1962–2018), head of secretariat Presidential Advisory Council on Ebola (PACE), posthumously; Ms. Miatta Gbanya, deputy incident manager for financial management; Dr. Francis Kateh, deputy incident manager for medical services; Mr. James Dorbor Jallah, deputy incident manager for support services; Mr. Thomas Nagbe, deputy incident manager for county coordination; Hon. C. Sanford Wesseh, assistant minister of health for vital statistics and head of contact tracing; Dr. Moses Massaquoi, head of case management; Dr. Thelma Nelson, head of infection prevention and control (IPC); Dr. Janice Cooper, head of psychosocial support; Dr. John Mulbah, Liberia Medical and Dental Council, ETU adviser; Mr. Mark Kovaryah, head of Dead Body Management team (DBM1); Mrs. Nadu Cooper, head, nutrition program; Ms. Siatta Bishop, (deceased 2022) head of crematorium (posthumously); Rev. John Sumo, head, social mobilization and community engagement; Mr. Luke Bawo, head, epidemiology and surveillance; Dr. Philip Sarh (from 2014 to 2015) and Mr. Heny Korha (2016), heads, National Reference Laboratory; Mr. Karsor Kollie, deputy chair IMS Montserrado County; Dr. Mosoka Fallah, head of Active Case Finding/Community Based-Initiative (CBI), and Mr. Sumo Nuworlo, assistant to Dr. Fallah; Dr. Stephen Kennedy, head of Ebola vaccine research; Dr. Fatoma Bolay, co-head of vaccine research (posthumously); Mr. Philip Bemah, deputy head, case management; Mr. Amos Gborie, EOC manager; Mr. Abraham Nyenswah, deputy EOC manager; Mr. Sonpon Sieh, Monterrado IMC chair; Dr. Yatta Wapoe, deputy Montserrado

County IMS chair; county health officers of Liberia's fifteen counties from 2014 to 2016; Ms. Elizabeth Kwemi, my assistant; and Mr. Jaygbah Mulbah, my able special assistant who worked with me tirelessly from start to end. I acknowledge the entire incident management support team and principal collaborating organizations, the Liberian health care workforce, the Liberian media, community volunteers, civil society organizations, and religious institutions for their role in kicking Ebola out of Liberia.

United Nations System: Thanks to H. E. Ban Ki-moon, former UN secretary-general; Dr. Margaret Chan, former director-general, WHO; Dr. David Nabarro, former special advisor to the UN secretary-general; Dr. Nestor Ndayimirije, former WHO representative; Dr. Alex Gasasira, former WHO representative; Mr. Peter Graaff, former head of the UN Mission on Ebola Emergency Response (UNMEER) in Liberia; Mr. Tony Banbery, former head of UNMEER regional office in Ghana; Dr. Antonio Virgilitti, former resident coordinator, UNDP, and deputy special representative to the secretary-general; Sheldon Yett, country representative, UNICEF; Dr. Remi Sogunro, UN Population Fund, World Food Programme, and UN Office of Project Services; Dr. Kamil Kayode Kamaluddeen, former UNDP representative to Liberia; Mrs. Inguna Dobraja, World Bank country manager to Liberia; Mr. Shunsuke Mabuchi, task team leader for the World Bank Emergency Response Project; and Dr. Munirat Iyabode Ayoka Ogunlayi, senior health officer of the World Bank in Liberia.

African Development Bank (AFDB): Mrs. Margaret Kilo, country manager to Liberia.

African Union: To all its member states that galvanized support for the Ebola response in West Africa, thank you for sending over one hundred medics, epidemiologists, and other public health professionals to assist us.

Economic Community of West African States: Special thanks to the government and people of the Federal Republic of Nigeria, as well as the Nigeria Centre for Disease Control—especially Professor Abdul-salami Nasidi, director-general—for rallying to the cause and sending the first team of medical personnel and epidemiologists to work with us in the field to stop transmission of Ebola in the region.

Government of the United States of America: Thanks to Deborah Malac, former US ambassador to Liberia; Dr. Tom Frieden, former director, US Centers for Disease Control and Prevention (CDC); Dr. Kevin De Cock, CDC Ebola Response Team lead to Liberia; Dr. Desmond Williams, former CDC country director to Liberia; Dr. Frank Mohaney, senior epidemiologist; Mr. Ed Rouse, CDC; Ms. Jana L. Telfer, CDC 2014 response health promotion team lead; to all the US government responders and organizations: Maj. Gen. Gary Volesky and Maj. Gen. Darryl Williams, DOD; USAID, OFDA, USPHS, and DHHS; and Drs. Anthony Fauci and H. Clifford Lane, National Institutes of Health, for their immense role in establishing the Ebola vaccines research and therapeutics in Liberia.

Government of the People's Republic of China: Thanks to Zhang Yue, the Chinese ambassador to Liberia and the Chinese Army for setting up and managing an Ebola treatment unit. Dr. George F. Gao, director-general Chinese Center for Disease Control and Prevention.

Government of the Republic of Cuba: Thanks to Uordenie Despaigne Vera, Chargé d'Affaires, and the team of fifty Cuban medical personnel who came in early and stayed throughout the response, without any fanfare.

Thanks to the following friends from educational institutions: Dr. Emmet Dennis (deceased 2022), former president of the University of Liberia, for his professional and fatherly advisory role to me; Dr. David Peters, former Edgar Berman chair, Department of International Health, Johns Hopkins Bloomberg School of Public Health, who supported Liberia's health management information system and recovery process; Dr. David C. Henderson, chairman of the Department of Psychiatry at Boston University School of Medicine (BUSM) and psychiatrist in chief at Boston Medical Center (BMC), for giving us office space and logistical support to write several sections of this book; Dr. Christina Borba, director, Office for Disparities Research and Workforce Diversity, National Institute of Mental Health; Dr. Paul Farmer, Harvard University, co-founder of Partners-in-Health (deceased 2022); Dr. Alison Galvani, director, Yale Center for Infectious Disease Modeling and Analysis, who seconded Dr. Laura Skrip, then PhD student from Yale University, to help with CBI and active case findings; Dr. Alison provided financial support, data analysis and modeling, and contributed laptop computers to support NPHIL's computer center; Mr. J. Stephen Morrison, senior vice president and director, Global Health Policy Center, Center for Strategic and International Study, for inviting me to speak at a forum in Washington, DC, and to share my Ebola experiences with the rest of the world.

Special thanks to Watchen and William Bruce, who provided us the space and time in their home when we worked together in Baltimore to restructure our second draft; and to Rev. Charles and Jurudoe Martin, who opened their home and gave us a quiet space to write and work with our first copyeditor.

Profound gratitude to Mr. Robin W. Coleman, acquisitions editor, Johns Hopkins University Press, for believing in me and supporting the development of this work. Without his confident and unflinching support, this book would not have been published today. Robin provided us with a developmental editor, Mojie Crigler, who worked with us on restructuring and editing the final draft of the manuscript. We thank her for her guidance and patience. The journey was long, but there was light at the end of the tunnel. I would also like to acknowledge Hyunjee Nicole Kim, the copy editor who assisted us in refining the style and flow of the content in the early stages. We also thank the reviewers of the initial and final manuscripts.

To Dr. Mardia Stone, my most able senior and technical advisor throughout the Ebola response up until now, I extend my profound gratitude. She encouraged me to write this book and assisted me in formulating my thoughts from its inception. This work was crafted with her guidance, support, and literary acumen through all of its various phases. She has worked with me assiduously to see it to fruition. Dr. Stone grasped what was at stake from the beginning and knew that other outbreaks were just a matter of time. She insisted that the Liberian story be told. She said, "Tolbert, others will write about the 2014–16 Ebola outbreak, but your story will be unique—the story that everybody will want to read—and no one can write it better than yourself."

Above all I bow my head before God Almighty, who has been my ultimate guide and has enabled me to write this book. Without Him, this would not have been possible.

We honor the memory of all those who lost their lives during the battle with the deadly Ebola virus in Liberia. My heart goes out to them each time I visit Disco Hill Cemetery on the Roberts International Airport Highway, where their bodies are laid to rest.

Collapse
and Resiliency

Introduction

On August 11, 2014, the Liberian minister of health, Dr. Walter T. Gwenigale, asked me into his office to say I'd been called to national duty by our president, Ellen Johnson Sirleaf. She wanted me to lead the national Ebola response as the incident manager. My reaction was absolute shock. *Why me?* I wondered to myself. *Why have I, a junior officer, been singled out for such a humongous task? Why not my bosses, the minister himself, or the chief medical officer, Dr. Bernice Dahn, who was my immediate supervisor? How would I be able to handle the biggest health crisis in the history of our country? Was it worth the risk of contracting Ebola and infecting my wife and young children?*

Despite all of these questions, I knew instinctively that I had to accept the responsibility and do all that was necessary to stop the spread of Ebola in our country. Although I was aware that the Ebola outbreak was already out of control, I recognized the honor of being selected to a unique leadership role in the wake of an unprecedented epidemic in our nation's history and the world at large. And I recognized that it was a dream my father had had the day I was born. He often told me when I was growing up that I was born to lead our nation someday. This was my destiny, he said.

So, with humility and resolve—and not fully understanding the magnitude of the task—I accepted the responsibility to serve as chairman of the Incident Management System (IMS) to fight the Ebola virus disease (EVD) outbreak in Liberia. It was a tremendous challenge, and I committed to serving my country to the best of my ability. When I returned home that evening, I went to my bedroom, changed my clothes, and knelt down to pray to God for guidance. I prayed for the wisdom to lead, I prayed for the wisdom to know who the right people were to help me, and I prayed that the best available health professionals in Liberia would emerge so that, collectively, we could accomplish the task of overcoming Ebola and preventing the decimation of our entire country.

As the Ebola epidemic in Liberia reached its peak, and the largest and most sustained Ebola outbreak ever was recorded, it became clear on the global front that the Ebola virus was cause for concern. The disease had spread from Liberia to Nigeria by an infected passenger who boarded a Nigerian airline to Lagos, the most populous city in the country. This began the secondary transmission of Ebola in the West African region. Back in Liberia, two American missionaries working in a missionary hospital run by Americans were diagnosed with EVD. They were evacuated to the United States, with much fanfare, after receiving experimental drugs brought in by doctors on the private air ambulance that came to get them. Ebola was no longer considered "an exotic tropical infection" but a highly infectious disease that could cross borders and impact health security. It then became a global health priority, prompting further heightened discussions on experimental drugs and the necessity of enhancing vaccine research and therapeutics during the active phase of the epidemic.

At the other end of the spectrum, Liberians demanded that their government require international organizations to outline clear evacuation policies for international staff exposed to or infected with EVD, particularly so because Liberian nationals working for the same international organizations did not get the same preferential treatment when exposed or infected. We were overwhelmed and overstretched as locally our capacity to handle the epidemic with regard to contact tracing and containment was not initially up to par and the epidemic escalated, far out of control, impeding Liberia's already weak health care system. There was complete closure or staff abandonment of hospitals with EVD cases nationwide. Many expatriates and Liberians who had the means fled the country in fear. Most airlines halted flights to Monrovia, the nation's capital, while those traveling out of Liberia were often refused entry into some countries. The US Centers for Disease Control and Prevention (CDC) warned Americans against unnecessary travel to West Africa. With the assistance of foreign partners, Liberians resolved to change the trend of the outbreak by intensifying response activities, changing strategic direction, and ultimately containing Ebola and halting the epidemic.

The EVD epidemic in Liberia made us aware that globally, we are all interconnected. We easily and in short time frames traverse continents and regional borders via air, land, or sea. The recognition of this interconnectedness underscores the commonalities and vulnerabilities of the easy access globalization affords us. In Liberia, we are now focused on integrated disease surveillance, emergency preparedness, and response in building a more resilient health care delivery system that is available and accessible to all, in every corner of the nation. Ebola taught us that every sector of the government has to work together in an emergency; the lessons we learned from this outbreak are integrated into all of our short- and long-term plans. By building a health care system that is resilient, available, and accessible to all our citizens, we created sustainable solutions to ensure that future catastrophic epidemics, such as Ebola, are prevented.

The turning point of Liberia's response efforts was President Sirleaf's message to citizens of Liberia, the West African Region, and the rest of the world. In her message, the president said:

> Since March, we have faced a terrible tragedy in our country. Along with our sister Republics of Guinea and Sierra Leone, we continue to battle an unprecedented outbreak of the Ebola virus disease. . . .

Our cultural and our family practices did not help when we finally woke up to the disease so we have to keep telling each other about what to do.

When a patient is sick with Ebola it is crucial that they are isolated from others and given appropriate care. But we know that for families to see their loved ones being taken where they are not able to follow and be with them is strange and frightening. We also know that to have a case of Ebola in a family can lead to stigma and shame. . . .

. . . We have lost mothers, fathers, sons and daughters. In some instances it has taken multiple members of families. . . .

The World Health Organization has declared the outbreak an international public health emergency. In the next few days, the Centers for Disease Control and Prevention will release projections about trajectory of the outbreak based on current trends and data. . . .

I want you, the Liberian people, to know that your government will do all that is within our power to ensure that the scenario in the projections do not come to pass. . . . We have enlisted the help of our bilateral and multilateral partners. We will continue to take clear actions and introduce the measures required to break the transmission chain and reverse the spread of the virus.

And you, our citizens[,] must do your part. . . . We will continue to ask for international help, but until we take responsibility of this problem as individuals, as families, as neighborhoods, as communities, as districts, as counties and as a nation, this problem will not go away.[1]

President Sirleaf was referring to a chilling projection modeling, she and I were briefed on by CDC that "between 550,000 and 1.4 million people could be infected by Ebola in the three most affected countries by January 20, 2015" if robust intervention were not put in place.[2]

After President Sirleaf's message, the United Nations, foreign governments, aid agencies, nongovernmental organizations, and private entities offered an outpouring of support—technical, financial, infrastructural, and humanitarian—and partnerships, which together turned things around and changed the course of the epidemic in Liberia.

Ebola Hits Liberia

The baby was sucking her mother's breast, but the mother had died from Ebola.

Can you fathom this?

When I saw them, I wondered, *Does the baby know her mother is dead, yet cannot let go?*

The woman had been dead for a while and was starting to decay, but still the baby clung to her. The baby's five-year-old sibling was there too, also holding onto their mother.

This mother's death occurred in Caldwell, a town on the outskirts of Monrovia. It was one of countless tragedies in the horror that was the West African Ebola epidemic. Between March 2014 and May 2016, over 28,000 people were infected and more than 11,300 people died, mainly in Guinea, Liberia, and Sierra Leone.[1] It is possible that the statistical data do not adequately reflect the magnitude of the outbreak.[2,3]

I pray that the souls of the dead rest in peace.

In Liberia, Ebola wreaked havoc on the fragile health care system, but the virus was not solely a medical problem. It crushed all aspects of normal life. The country's borders were closed. Schools were shuttered. Those who lived did so with unrelenting fear, which often turned into anger and panic.

This is my story of the Ebola crisis: how the virus broke Liberia and how the country survived and rebuilt itself. This is also the story of my own journey, from a village to my time as a refugee and, ultimately, my leadership of Liberia's Ebola response. I offer these stories as lessons of good and bad practices—in honor of those who died, as a tribute to those who helped, and as a somber warning to the world that this should never happen again.

In early March 2014, news reached the Ministry of Health and Social Welfare (MOHSW) that a severe disease outbreak had started in Guinea, near the Liberian border, in a town called Meliandou in Gueckedou Prefecture. A two-year-old boy had died in December 2013. The boy, later identified as Emile Ouamouno, became known as the first, or index, case of the West African Ebola epidemic.[4] His mother, sister, and grandmother then became ill with similar symptoms and also died. People infected by those initial cases spread the disease to other villages. Although Ebola represents a major public health threat in sub-Saharan Africa, no cases had ever been reported in West Africa and the early cases were misdiagnosed as other diseases more common to the area. Thus, Ebola had several months to spread before it was recognized.[5,6]

At the time, I was assistant minister and deputy chief medical officer (CMO) for preventive services at the MOHSW. At the ministry and as a citizen, I was not alone in thinking, at first, that the outbreak sounded so far away. Surely it would never reach Liberia, and certainly not the capital, Monrovia. I had lived in Monrovia since 1997; in early 2014, life in the city felt normal. But on March 30, authorities at the MOHSW notified the World Health Organization (WHO) that the first Ebola case had been confirmed in Liberia.[7]

Reporting Ebola was an obligation by member states of WHO as a fulfilment of the International Health Regulations (IHR) of 2005. The IHR, first adopted by the World Health Assembly in 1969 and last revised in 2005, are a legally binding instrument of international law that aims for international cooperation to "prevent, protect against, control and provide a public health response to the international spread of disease in ways that are commensurate with and restricted to public health risks and that avoid unnecessary interference with international traffic and trade."[8,9] The IHR are the only international legal treaty with the responsibility of empowering the WHO to act as the main global surveillance system.[10,11]

Liberia's index case, in late March 2014, was the result of cross-border transmission by an infected person from Guinea, who was believed to have visited relatives in the town of Foya in Lofa County, Liberia. It is assumed that relatives who came into direct contact with the diseased in Foya also became infected and died. Then, several infected people, without symptoms, traveled from Foya to Monrovia in commercial vehicles. Commercial transport vehicles in rural Lofa County are often overcrowded. The journey to Monrovia could take nine hours or longer given the poor road conditions at that time, and cars or minibuses did not always cover the full distance. Passengers usually had to change vehicles at various transit points before reaching their final destination. Unwitting passengers were exposed to a sick passenger, practically sitting on top each other in a tight taxi, bus, or pickup truck. By the end of the journey, the virus had been transmitted. By late March, the disease had hit Monrovia.

Thus, the madness of Ebola in Liberia began.

Ebola virus disease (EVD) is a rare and deadly disease in people and nonhuman primates (e.g., monkeys, baboons, and apes).[12] The viruses that cause EVD are located mainly in sub-Saharan Africa. People can get EVD through direct contact with an infected animal, person, or corpse.[12] In Liberia, infections mostly occurred while performing funeral rituals and unsafe burial practices.[13]

At the time of the outbreak in West Africa, there was no approved vaccine or treatment for EVD. Research focused on finding the virus's natural host, developing vaccines to protect at-risk populations, and discovering therapies to improve treatment of the disease.[14] EVD had been discovered in 1976 in two simultaneous outbreaks, one in what is now Nzara, South Sudan, and the other in Yambuku, Democratic Republic of Congo, in a village near the Ebola River, which gave the disease its name.[12]

Ebola comes from a family of viruses called *Filoviridae*. There are three types, or genera, of *Filoviridae*: *Cuevavirus*, *Marburgvirus*, and *Ebolavirus*.[12] Within the genus *Ebolavirus*, five species have been identified: Bundibugyo, Zaire, Sudan, Reston, and Taï Forest.[12] Of these, *Bundibugyo ebolavirus*, *Zaire ebolavirus*, and *Sudan ebolavirus* have been associated with large outbreaks in Africa.[12,15] The *Zaire ebolavirus* species was the cause of the 2014–2016 West African outbreak, which was the first widespread Ebola outbreak in West Africa since the disease first surfaced in 1976.[15,16] It was also the largest and most complex Ebola outbreak ever, with three times more reported cases and deaths than all other previous outbreaks combined, and which crossed national and international borders. Whereas the first outbreaks occurred in remote villages near tropical rainforests in Eastern and Central Africa, the West African outbreak involved rural and urban areas, including the capital cities of the three most affected countries.

EVD was once known as Ebola fever, or viral hemorrhagic fever, because it affects all major systems in the body and causes an infected person to bleed from practically every orifice. This severe hemorrhaging usually results in a person bleeding to death. While no cure exists, survival improves with supportive care, rehydration, and symptomatic treatment soon after symptoms appear. Although there is as yet no licensed treatment proven to neutralize the virus, a range of blood, immunological, and drug therapies are under development. The average EVD case fatality rate is around 50%. Case fatality rates have ranged from 25% to 90% in past outbreaks.[17]

Symptoms of EVD usually occur within two to twenty-one days after a person has direct contact with the virus. Most infected individuals will manifest symptoms within this incubation period, with the average being eight to ten days after exposure.[18] Common symptoms include a high and unrelenting fever, severe or pounding headache, generalized weakness, fatigue, muscular pain, severe persistent diarrhea, excessive vomiting, stomach aches (abdominal pain), and incessant bleeding or bruising (unexplained hemorrhage) from the mouth, ears, eyes, nose, and/or anus.[18] Some Ebola symptoms are similar to those of common illnesses, such as influenza, malaria, and Lassa fever.

People may recover from EVD if they have a strong immune system response and if they receive good supportive care and treatment based on signs and symptoms at the onset. Researchers following those fortunate enough to survive EVD have found that antibodies (molecules made by the immune system to attack and destroy invading pathogens) remain in the blood up to ten years after recovery.[19]

In Guinea, before mid-April 2014, there were 168 cases and 108 deaths in six prefectures, according to the WHO.[20] Infections then spread to Conakry, the capital. Meanwhile, cases in Lofa were increasing. Lofa had the highest concentration of Ebola infections in Liberia, as more Guineans crossed the border into Lofa.[20] By late April 2014, Liberia reported 35 cases, mostly in Foya, while Guinea then had 218 cases and 141 deaths.[13,20] The Lofa County health team responded to the outbreak, supported by a team dispatched from Monrovia and headed by Thomas Nagbe, director of MOHSW's Disease Prevention Division (DPC). In Foya, the team set up the first Ebola isolation unit, for fewer than ten people, but they were handicapped due to logistics. Lacking a car, they transported Ebola samples by canoe across the river into Guinea. It would take weeks, if not months, for the results to be known.

In May 2014, the first EVD case in Sierra Leone was reported in Kailahun District, which shares borders with Guinea and Liberia; EVD spread to neighboring Kenema District in June 2014.[21] Cases escalated quickly, a factor of cross-border migration between Sierra Leone, Guinea, and Liberia. The borders are extremely porous, and populations are highly mobile. Even though there are boundary lines and immigration checkpoints at border crossings, numerous footpaths wind through forests and are not manned by officials. Families live on both sides of the border. In the early stages of the epidemic, it was extremely difficult to track people who may have been exposed to Ebola.

Sierra Leone, like Guinea and Liberia, had no experience dealing with Ebola. Compounding the problem, each nation had a very fragile health care system. Each was a post-conflict nation. What the disease is and how it is transmitted was an ongoing pursuit. Public health officials knew what Ebola was only from textbooks and studying public health and medicine. The general population knew little about what Ebola was. Varying perceptions and misperceptions depended on regional differences. Ebola's control measures were unknown except that it killed people quickly, in a matter of days, and there was no cure. Death could come merely through touching or coming close to an infected person. The death rate was high, and an Ebola death was absolutely horrific: bleeding from everywhere, vomiting, everything coming out from below, running like a red river—bloody diarrhea, bloody urine, bloody sweat, even bloody tears. Fever would be so high that a person could burn and sweat with their head pounding. Those infected didn't stand a chance; they would be dead within weeks, even days. What a fate!

The context in which the outbreak occurred contributed significantly to the escalation. Liberia ranks 175 out of 187 countries in human development.[22] The gross domestic product (GDP) per capita was last reported in 2019 at US$1,427.80. The GDP per capita in Liberia, when adjusted by purchasing power parity, is equivalent to 8% of the world's average.[23] With 64% of the population living in poverty, around 48% of the population is below the extreme poverty line. Prior to the Ebola outbreak in early 2014, Liberia was experiencing a period of rapid economic growth at an estimated 8.1%.[23]

The literacy rate is around 52% for women and 75% for men, age 15–49.[24] Urban Liberians are more likely than their rural counterparts to be literate. Sixty-three percent of urban women and 84% of urban men are literate, as compared with 34% of rural women and 61% of rural men.[24] Between 1989 and 2003, Liberia was engulfed in a civil conflict. The first war lasted from 1989 to 1997, and the second from 1999 to

2003.[25] A quarter million civilians were killed in the first civil war, about 60,000 in the second.[25,26,27]

Liberia's population is about 5 million. The southeast, toward Côte d'Ivoire, is less densely populated and harder to reach than the rest of the country. The country is divided into fifteen counties, with Montserrado County predominantly represented by the city of Monrovia.

Monrovia is congested; it is home to about 1.5 million people,[24] roughly one-third of Liberia's population. It has many overcrowded slums with inadequate housing and poor sanitation. Toilet facilities are nonexistent in many areas there, and people urinate and defecate in places that they find convenient. Some even relieve themselves in plastic bags, filling them with feces. These bags are known as "flying toilets" because they are often thrown in the air, aimed at a landing site, usually on top of piles of garbage or over fences, onto other people's property.

In April and most of May 2014, no new cases were reported in Liberia.[28] But the disease was there, spreading within households shared by family members who knew nothing about Ebola. Some became infected when preparing the dead for traditional burial. Others became infected when they sought care in a hospital; in health care settings, infection prevention and control were barely practiced if at all.

For example, in New Kru Town, a densely populated slum community just outside of central Monrovia, sick or injured people would go to Redemption Hospital, a government-run hospital in Montserrado County, which has the largest population density of all of Liberia's fifteen counties. Redemption Hospital was ill-equipped and understaffed to handle the influx of patients with varying degrees of acute and chronic illnesses unrelated to Ebola. There was a dearth of beds and space. General supplies were inadequate. The quality of care on a good day was questionable. Infection prevention was not always practiced—the hospital staff had no personal protective equipment (PPE) to keep them safe from contamination if they handled a patient displaying signs and symptoms of Ebola. Redemption also had no designated isolation unit in which to quarantine patients suspected of having Ebola. There was nowhere to take the gravely ill for supportive care and treatment.

By late July, there were only two 20-bed Ebola treatment units (ETUs) in the entire country.[28] One of these ETUs was at the ELWA Hospital, in Paynesville, a little over fifteen miles from central Monrovia. ELWA (Eternal Love Winning Africa), the entity, was established in 1951 by Serving in Mission (SIM), a Christian organization. ELWA Hospital sits on a 130-acre site loaned by the Liberian government for the expressed purpose of building a school and hospital, providing services that would benefit Liberians. The hospital expanded and a school was built, however most of the land was still undeveloped. In the 1950s, supported by Samaritan's Purse, a missionary organization headquartered in the United States, ELWA began with a radio station and a small hospital. When Ebola hit, Dr. Jerry Brown, a trained Liberian surgeon and medical director of the ELWA Hospital, sealed off the hospital's chapel as an isolation and treatment area for patients suspected of having Ebola, after consultation with Dr. Bernice Dahn, the deputy minister of health services/chief medical officer of Liberia. The chapel was small and not conducive to patient care, but it became a makeshift ETU that could hold a limited number of patients. Dr. Brown convinced some of his nursing and ancillary staff to work with him in the ETU.

In the coming months, ELWA Hospital was forced to turn people away due to lack of space and adequate staffing. Many people became angry and threatened Dr. Brown and his staff. Being the compassionate doctor that he is, and in his wisdom as medical director, Dr. Brown converted a laundry room behind the hospital into an additional ETU and named it ELWA 2. With a bed capacity of no more than fifty beds, it would not be enough to handle the overwhelming number of Ebola patients.

The initial stages of the MOHSW's response focused primarily on providing curative medicine in areas where transmission rates were high. Without truly knowing or understanding what we were confronting, we employed control measures that had proven to be effective in Ebola outbreaks in other countries, such as the Democratic Republic of the Congo (DRC), previously known as Zaire, and Uganda. However, in those settings they had never seen an Ebola outbreak of this magnitude. Essential health services, already degraded prior to the outbreak, were neglected, mainly because health care workers feared for their lives and refused to go to work due to a lack of personal protective equipment or other necessary items to protect them from getting infected. Infection prevention and control measures were not in place; where they may have existed, they were not practiced. Poor infection control measures and practices led to high infection rates among health care workers. Much to their dismay, health care workers did not receive expected incentives or hazard pay from the government to motivate them to get involved in the Ebola response. Consequently, they went on strike to express their displeasure.

At the onset of the Ebola epidemic, Liberia had fifty medical doctors for its entire population of 5 million.[29] There were only a few laboratories, which delayed sample collection and reporting results. Consequently, interventions were not immediate and case management was hindered. Data management (epidemiological surveillance) was exceptionally poor. There were only two public health laboratory scientists and three PhD-level biomedical scientists. The country's only dedicated medical research campus, consisting of the Liberia Institute of Biomedical Research (LIBR) and the National Reference Laboratory (NRL), had serious capacity issues. There were not enough trained staff to manage diagnostic needs and investigate therapeutic or prophylactic targets. These disabling circumstances delayed confirmatory diagnosis of Ebola, as samples had to be taken to Guinea, Senegal, or Europe. This contributed to the prolonged spread of the Ebola virus in Liberia. Additionally, the dysfunction of the health care system during the epidemic resulted in the closure of facilities that were providing non-Ebola routine care, resulting in yet another emergency during the outbreak. Several hundred health care workers became infected and died, including Liberia's only two internists.[30]

By July, Monrovia reeked of dead bodies. People afraid of getting Ebola were throwing dead bodies in the streets—often the sick were left to die there. The stench and sights were unbearable. Sick people were languishing in communities across Monrovia and the nearby counties of Margibi, Bomi, and Grand Cape Mount.

Liberians felt that the government was not earnest about combating the disease and voiced their opinions. There was agitation in the streets; citizens called for the government to resign and that President Sirleaf should step down and turn the response over to the international community. Opposition politicians accused the government of doing little or nothing to halt the outbreak. By not engaging the community initially, social mobilization and sensitization campaigns were ineffective and most likely enabled disease transmission. The complexities of the Ebola epidemic clearly posed a threat to political incumbents and the political system at large. The airwaves were saturated with conflicting messages. These messages needed to be properly aligned with the government's overall public health messages, but they were not. The public grew more convinced that the government did not know what to do. The government's approach was to wait and see what the donors—that is, other countries and international aid organizations—would bring or give. Hence, the response structure going forward was heavily donor dependent.

The international response came slowly. Médecins Sans Frontières (MSF; Doctors Without Borders), which had been responding to the outbreak in Guinea, warned that the epidemic could be unprecedented in size. The warning fell on deaf ears.[31] The World Health Organization broadcast conflicting messages, first saying that the outbreak was small, then, in mid-April, voicing alarm.[31]

In July, only MSF, WHO, and the United States Agency for International Development (USAID) were supporting the MOHSW. They already had country representatives. WHO is the lead technical partner agency in Liberia, USAID had been in Liberia for decades, and MSF-Belgium had been in Liberia since the civil war, providing humanitarian services and running clinics and hospitals in Monrovia. When Ebola struck, MSF-Belgium was invited to join Liberia's response by Dr. Dahn, then chief medical officer. Dr. Dahn had been persuaded to extend this invitation by Dr. Moses Massaquoi, a member of MSF's board of directors as well as country director for the Clinton Foundation / Clinton Health Access Initiative.

MSF made an agreement with the Ministry of Health to set up an ETU with about twenty to twenty-five beds. The equipment had to be imported from France, and it took about ten days to arrive. MSF began setting up the prefabricated ETU on vacant land on the ELWA compound, a distance from the hospital. The International Federation of Red Cross (IFRC) also arrived and, with the Liberian Red Cross, started to help manage dead bodies.

On July 16, a seven-member team from the US Centers for Disease Control and Prevention (CDC) arrived in Monrovia to assess the extent of Liberia's preparedness to manage the response.[13] The team was led by infectious disease epidemiologist Dr. Kevin De Cock. Their initial investigations focused on determining the extent and magnitude of the outbreak, including among health care workers; clarifying and strengthening data systems and reporting; coordinating enhancement of laboratory capacity; and providing overall support for the Liberian response, which at that point lacked coherence and organization.

Despite these actions by MSF, WHO, USAID, and the CDC, the situation worsened. In late July, the government ordered schools to be shut down to prevent widespread infection among students and staff. Official borders between Guinea and Liberia were closed, though there were numerous foot paths in the forest and people crossed the border anyway.

On July 27, President Ellen Johnson Sirleaf established the Presidential Task Force on Ebola, which she chaired. The president, I believed, was advised that Ebola was a national security crisis so as head of state she needed to be directly involved. The government had set up a diverse Ebola Task Force in March, headed by Minister of Health Dr. Walter

Gwenigale, with meetings usually chaired by Dr. Dahn, his deputy minister of health services, who also served as chief medical officer of Liberia. The large size of the Ebola Task Force and organizational challenges handicapped its effectiveness.

The Presidential Task Force was also impaired by its size and complex organizational structure. It consisted of the speaker of the House of Representatives, Hon. Alex Tyler, and members of the legislature, and the president's cabinet, including the minister of health and social welfare, the chief medical officer, the minister of defense, the minister of justice, the minister of internal affairs, the minister of information, inspector general of police, chief of the Bureau of Immigration and Naturalization, the national security advisor, as well as other senior government officials. Members of the interreligious council, comprising the Liberian Council of Churches, the Muslim Council, and the national traditional leaders, were also included.

According to my boss, Dr. Dahn, the main issues for discussion were the state of national confusion and the extent of the Ebola situation. All sorts of opinions were expressed, I understand, with some heated debates at times. Some officials suggested that a dusk-to-dawn curfew be imposed. What they seemed not to realize was that decisions from those early meetings did not help to stop Ebola from spreading. In fact, Ebola benefited from the state of anarchy and confusion.

Meanwhile, the logistics and financial management team was also meeting. Among their responsibilities was overseeing a national trust fund, which had been established by the president and approved by the national legislature with an initial amount of US$15 million.

A third group, the technical group, was assigned to follow the disease pattern and gauge the number of actual Ebola cases and the rate at which they occurred, as well as the number of people dying. As assistant minister and deputy chief medical officer for preventive services, I was in this group, along with Minister of Health Dr. Gwenigale, Deputy Minister for Health Services and CMO Dr. Dahn, MSF, USAID, WHO (through its country representative, Dr. Nestor Ndayimirije), and Samaritan's Purse.

The three groups did not talk to each other. Decisions made by one group were not shared with the others. Furthermore, the groups were physically spread out, working in different locations in Monrovia. The group that dealt with the medical aspects of the response operated from the Ministry of Health building in an area known as Congo Town, on the outskirts of central Monrovia. The logistics team was located across town in central Monrovia, in the offices of the General Services Agency, which managed government properties. This fragmentation resulted in different groups of people having independent meetings all over the place. Coordination was demonstrably poor. It was total chaos, and more people died every day.

I was never invited to provide any input during any of these meetings. In the high-level meeting chaired by the president, this was not surprising. I was a very junior member in the ministerial hierarchy. As an assistant minister, I reported to the CMO, who reported to the minister of health, who reported to the president. Because of my extensive education in public health, disease control and prevention, health administration, policy, and the law, I brought a wealth of knowledge to the issues. As the head of the Division of Disease Prevention, I was in charge of twenty-one disease control programs. Prior to my current post, I had successfully led programs on malaria, tuberculosis, HIV/ AIDS (human immunodeficiency virus/acquired immunodeficiency syndrome), maternal and child health, immunizations, and motorcycle safety. I held a master's degree in public health from the Johns Hopkins Bloomberg School of Public Health, Department of International Health. I had earned postgraduate certificates in global public health, human rights, epidemiology, and public health surveillance. I also had a degree in law from the University of Liberia. I could have given valuable opinions and recommendations, but the minister of health barred me from speaking each time meetings were held at the ministry. This was not unique to the minister of health—it's a pattern in the Liberian government due to the bureaucratic and hierarchical nature of the system. For example, I made recommendations to open the Island Clinic to create more bed space at a time when treatment beds were in acute shortage. I suggested we hire community health workers to do contact tracing, as we had with polio eradication community vaccination campaigns. These, among other suggestions, were ignored.

I was put in charge of the Social Mobilization (Social Mob) and Media Relations subcommittee. Reverend John Sumo, director of the Health Promotion Division, worked with me as the technical person. We were responsible for the entire communication strategy. Our messages became national slogans: Don't Touch! No Hugging! No Kissing! No Shaking Hands! No Eating Something! (This last admonition meant: no sex.) "No Touching!" practically became a salutation. Every day, everywhere, everyone resounded the message unapologetically: "No Touching!" In a nation where people snap fingers intertwined in a handshake and touch or hug more often than some would like, No Touching! was hard to do.

I was moving from one radio station to another, talking about Ebola, educating the public on Ebola, and making people aware of signs and symptoms and how to protect themselves. I went to nearly all government ministries and agencies with the same message. Our team fielded questions about Ebola prevention and control measures from the ministries and agencies in town hall–like meetings. A similar strategy would be used in communities that mobilized themselves across Monrovia and nearby counties.

Our Social Mob team went from community to community, making all efforts to engage community residents in the education and awareness campaign and to rally people for the cause. My crusade extended to media outlets around the world, including the BBC, CNN, the *New York Times*, the *Washington Post*, and Al Jazeera.

We were fighting two uphill battles: one against Ebola, the other against misinformation. Both had a head start.

Ebola affected people in ways they never imagined. Human interactions were put to a test on all scales. Families accustomed to showing affection were deterred. The No Touching! message hit home hard. No one was touching anyone. Even married people were mindful of No Touching!; everyone was cautious. People were suspicious of each other.

Relationships were strained. Marriages were no exception. Some believed that there would be a substantial economic collapse, that trading with long-established partners would suffer and foreign companies with enduring business relationships with the government would pack up and leave in order to save their companies and employees from Ebola. Folks were irritable, frustrated, and afraid. Ebola was spreading like wildfire and killing everyone in its path. It didn't spare caregivers who unknowingly had direct contact while caring for loved ones, nor did it spare health care professionals, who took oaths to provide care to the sick to the best of their ability and without distinction. Ebola spared no parent, child, brother, or sister who had direct contact with each other, simply living together as they normally would.

Everyone was at risk of contracting the uncompromisingly deadly disease, and people grew more terrified. No one wanted to die. The sense of doom was overwhelming.

CHAPTER 2

Born for Such a Time

My own story begins in a very different place.

I was born on September 10, 1974, in Panama, a remote rural village in Sinoe County, situated in the southeastern region of Liberia. Panama at the time had a population of less than 2,000 people. My parents are Ruth Tanneh Moses Nyenswah (alive) and Rev. William K. Moses Nyenswah (deceased), a Methodist pastor who was also an elementary school teacher. They named me Tolbert after Liberia's twenty-first president, William R. Tolbert Jr., who was also a Baptist preacher, and one whom my father greatly admired. The slogan of the Tolbert administration was "total involvement for higher heights." Tolbert's plan was embraced by people around the country, particularly after twenty-seven years of the administration of William V. S. Tubman, standard-bearer of the True Whig Party, under whom Tolbert had served as the vice president.

Although President Tubman was beloved by the people for his political savvy and American-style government and social leanings, he was also admired for his kind, caring, and giving nature. He shared his personal good fortune and that of the nation with family and friends alike. He educated people, gave them food, hired them directly, or ensured that they were gainfully employed. President Tubman initiated the National Unification Policy to bring all of Liberia's people together. He declared National Unification Day a public holiday, which is still celebrated every year on May 14. The benefactors of President Tubman's generosity spanned several generations. However, his prolonged tenure of twenty-seven years in office was questioned by the masses, who were mostly illiterate and poor, living in rural villages far removed from the fanfare of Tubman's government.

When President Tubman died in office in 1971, Tolbert ascended to the presidency. It was a welcome change. Tolbert's slogan, "total involvement for higher heights," meant that whether "civilized" (as elite and educated Liberians often referred to themselves) or "native" (as the villagers, townspeople, and the uneducated were called by the so-called civilized), everyone had to be involved in nation-building in every aspect to raise Liberia to the "higher heights" he envisioned. Tolbert made his government officials report to work at 8 a.m. sharp instead of whenever they got there, as was the typical practice during Tubman's time. He emphasized accountability. He led by example, and he traveled the country by road to remote areas like Panama, where my father had the rare privilege of meeting and hosting him. My father was so in awe of this man that when I was born, he saw in me the visions of President Tolbert, and thus blessed me with the first name Tolbert to honor the one he perceived to be a great statesman. Each time I attempted to change the spelling of my name to the Kru tribe name Torbor, it was to my father's displeasure. Sometimes I got a beating for that! He would tell me to spell my name the way Tolbert spelled his.

President Tolbert advocated a fixed eight-year term limit without the possibility of reelection for the president, instead of the four-year term without limits that was then allowed by the constitution. Many political elites vehemently opposed this reform. Tolbert became unpopular because of his many strict governmental rules, which he personally ensured were implemented. There were several demonstrations by young professionals, known as the "progressives," who opposed Tolbert's policies and politics.

In his book *Rich Land Poor Country: The "Paradox of Poverty" in Liberia*, Samuel P. Jackson,[1] who identifies himself as a member of the progressives, indicates that the progressives had the power to mobilize the public to act.[1] He says that the "Progressives were not an amorphous group of Liberians, yet the appellation stuck to nearly anyone who had ever expressed dissent against the government, including friends of the dissenters."[1] Jackson describes why, and how, university students became agitators against the Tolbert government. He posits that when President Tolbert's brother, Stephen Tolbert Sr. (Steve, as he was commonly called), sued Albert Porte, a renown pamphleteer, the progressives rose to his defense. Steve, who was also appointed the minister of finance by his brother, sued Porte because he reported extensively in his pamphlet on the "acquisition of the Sinoe Rubber Company from German investors," referring to the company's acquisition as "Gobbling Business."[1] There was a court judgment of US$250,000 against Porte for libel. The case later ended up at the Honorable Supreme Court and the Court upheld the $250,000 judgment against Porte.[1] According to Jackson, "the Tolbert Administration was being bombarded on all fronts, and its patience was wearing thin with the surge in agitation."[1] Young progressives became irate and vowed to organize protests in every possible manner, whenever, wherever, and however they could. They openly expressed their grievances against the Supreme Court's validation of the judgment against Albert Porte, as well as the president's reform policies, inter alia. The ability to openly protest was a new phenomenon. It was a "newfound freedom," widely embraced by students in secondary schools, universities, "labor unions, and civil society groups."[1] This broad-based agitation against Tolbert and his government escalated in 1975.[1]

On April 14, 1979, there was a mass riot against the increase in the price of a hundred-pound bag of rice, which soared from US$22 to $30. Rice is a staple food for Liberians, even though they do not grow enough to feed the country's population. Rice was imported in 1979, as it still is today. Given the price increase and the low wages of common folks, people took to the streets to get the president's attention. Tolbert, in his fury, ordered the military to quell what became known as the Rice Riot. The army moved aggressively into the crowds with heavy artillery and gunfire. Many people were murdered. Young progressives, students from the University of Liberia, and the poor were killed en masse—their dead bodies strewed all over the streets of Monrovia. A number of the political elites lost their children and other loved ones. The impoverished and common people lost the breadwinners of their families, many of whom worked as drivers, cooks, servants, and low-wage government employees. Then, upon the directives of the president, the government ordered the army to clear the corpses from the streets and dump them into a mass grave. The citizens were outraged. Those who mourned their dead relatives were even more furious, because it meant that the government's decision denied them the opportunity to give their cherished ones a dignified burial and peaceful rest, in a place they could visit whenever they wanted to ease their aching hearts. This made Tolbert more unpopular, mainly in Monrovia, the seat of government. Back in rural villages like Panama, my hometown, where news from Monrovia came rarely, Tolbert was still our beloved leader.

On April 12, 1980, one year after the Rice Riot, President Tolbert was murdered execution-style in the presidential residence of the Executive Mansion on Capitol Hill during the coup d'état that toppled his government. It is said that he was disemboweled and beheaded by Master Sergeant Samuel Kanyon Doe of the Liberian army, who was named the assassin and perceived to have led the coup. However, there are conflicting stories as to who the real coup plotters were and who actually assassinated the president. Many soldiers serving in the armed forces of Liberia at that time were usually not educated or only functionally literate and perceived not to be clever enough to successfully execute a coup. Or so we thought. Therefore, the general population felt that it was inconceivable that the low-ranking soldiers who claimed to have assassinated Mr. Tolbert actually killed him.

There were those who alleged that the US government had a hand in overthrowing the government and assassinating the president, using low-ranking soldiers as the front men. Tolbert was a bold and dynamic visionary. After twenty-seven years as Tubman's vice president, he made decisions and policies very distinct from Mr. Tubman's leanings toward the US involvement in Liberia's political and economic progression. He was resistant to the continuing influence of the US government in the affairs of Liberia and was more daringly inclined toward fostering diplomatic and other relationships with the Union of Soviet Socialist Republics (USSR) and the People's Republic of China.[2] His courage to tread new paths transformed the US-fashioned liberal capitalism to an industrialized, state capitalistic economic system, by establishing over thirty state-owned enterprises and concentrating on agriculture development, with the intent of making Liberia the producer of its own food. He wanted the country to be self-sufficient in every aspect. With this goal planted in the minds of Liberians ("total involvement for higher heights"), the government imposed restrictions on the facilities operated by the US military in Liberia.[2] Agreements previously signed with several major foreign companies, such as Firestone during the Tubman era, were renegotiated.[2] These bold moves in the interest of his country are what, many elites believed, led to the beginning of President Tolbert's downfall.

Tolbert's government was considered to be very progressive in advocating for "pan-African unity against neo-colonialism and promoted the Declaration on the Establishment of a New International Economic Order, adopted by the UN General Assembly in 1974."[2] Tolbert also was engaged in constructing the Monrovia Declaration, which was adopted in 1979 by the Organization of African Unity (OAU, now African Union [AU]) at its meeting hosted by Liberia.[3] The Lagos Plan of Action for Economic Development of Africa, 1980–2000, was derived from this declaration. The Lagos Plan of Action specifically states that "the exploitation of Africa continued to be carried out through neo-colonialist external forces which seek to influence the economic policies and directions of the African States,"[3,4] contrary to the 1981 World Bank's Berg Report and its structural adjustment programs for Africa.[4,5,6]

As is characteristic whenever leaders in non-western countries on any continent make firm economic and political decisions or transform the status quo from foreign political influence and economic dominance in their countries, there is often covert western interreference to change the regimes. We've seen this way too often in Africa. In the case of Mr. Tolbert, it is believed that the US Central Intelligence Agency (CIA) supported opposition groups to create more agitation. One such group was the Progressive Alliance of Liberia (PAL), headed by the late Gabriel Baccus Matthews.[5,6,7] On April 14, 1979, PAL led a massive protest in Monrovia against the government's national plan to boost domestic rice production toward food security and self-sufficiency by increasing taxes on imported rice. PAL publicly declared that this tax increase and the resulting inflation in the price of rice to the local consumer was a profit-making effort favoring rice importers and Mr. Tolbert's own business in rice production. The demonstration resulted in the Rice Riot, violent exchanges between the protesters and armed security forces firing on the crowds.[7] The government of Liberia firmly believed that the Rice Riot was due to foreign interference. About six months after the Rice Riot, a supposed confidential memorandum surfaced from the White House, in which was conveyed that, because of the riot in Monrovia "it was unlikely Tolbert would survive until the end of his term in 1983."[7] On April 12, 1980, President Tolbert was shot and savagely disemboweled at the Executive Mansion by seventeen armed noncommissioned soldiers in Liberia's army. "One of the soldiers, Albert Toe, recalls that after having killed Tolbert, the coup makers contacted the US Embassy, which endorsed the coup and promised to provide all necessary support."[7] Samuel Kanyon Doe, a master sergeant, was the highest-ranking officer, who claimed to have led the coup. He made the announcement on national radio that a military coup had taken place and that a military junta, under the name of the People's Redemption Council (PRC), had taken power under his leadership.[7]

Several military officials and generals in the mansion died in the gunfire and fighting. They were buried in a mass grave with the president at Palm Grove Cemetery on Center Street in Monrovia. Shortly afterward, the PRC began searching for his cabinet ministers. Those who got wind of the plan got away; thirteen, however, were found in their homes, offices, or other locations. They were brought to a central location at the military barracks in Monrovia. Ten days after the president's murder, these thirteen men, who were considered his trusted officials, were taken to an area of the beach known as South Beach. Each was stripped naked and tied to a log pole. Crowds of people flocked to the beach to see the spectacle for themselves. Many had never seen these men up close or even knew their names. They only knew that they were supposedly "big shots" who had been stripped of their fancy clothes and left naked for all to see and ridicule. Their only crime was that they had served their country under a man who was once adored and then hated. As the crowd booed, the naked men, strapped to log poles, were shot by a firing squad with multiple rounds of ammunition on command of the army, until they died. Their lifeless bodies were removed amid the cheers of the crowd and loaded in a dump truck. Their corpses were taken to Palm Grove Cemetery and buried in a mass grave, like the president, his generals, and the many victims of the Rice Riot. Master Sergeant Samuel Kanyon Doe of the Liberian army, Tolbert's named assassin, became head of state, commander in chief of the armed forces of Liberia.

My middle name, Geewleh, denotes a lion. My surname, Nyenswah, means God in the Kru language. The Kru is one of Liberia's sixteen indigenous tribes. From the day I was born, my parents believed that I, Tolbert Geewleh Nyenswah, was destined to lead our country. My dad always told me that one day I would save my tribe, my county, my community, my country, and ultimately the entire world. He said he was grooming me for a leadership role, which he was certain would manifest before I turned forty. As a child, I did not know or understand exactly what he meant.

My father, a Methodist pastor, was a public-school teacher employed by the government. His work gave our family the stability to keep a permanent home. Born in 1932 as the son of a paramount chief, he rose to become the acting district superintendent for the Methodist Church,

Sinoe District Conference. My father was a very handsome man: tall in stature with a well-developed physique and a broad face with small, deep-set eyes, a mocha complexion, and an inviting smile. He was a polygamist, as culture and tradition dictated at the time. My mother, Ruth, was his first, or head, wife. Together they had six children: three girls and three boys. I am the third child and second boy. A traditional village midwife delivered most of us at home, including me. Others were delivered in local health facilities.

Papa, as we called him, took a second wife, Martha, who bore him two sons, but for mysterious reasons Martha did not remain long in our household. One day she moved out with her two children. Yet they remained constant in our lives and after a year or so the children returned to live with us. My mother raised all eight children together as her own.

As my mother grew older and as native laws and customs allowed, she found my father another wife, a younger, prettier, and physically stronger girl named Suzanna. My dad, in agreement, paid Suzanna's dowry to her family and married her when she was just fourteen years old. She became his third wife. It was acceptable and common in traditional polygamous societies that older men marry girls, in some instances as young as twelve. Men could have as many wives as they could afford. One motive was to have as many children by their numerous wives to provide labor for farming and other pursuits. In addition to my mother's six children and Martha's two sons, Suzanna had seven children, making a total of fifteen Nyenswah children living together in one household. My father never showed any difference toward us as his children. He treated each of us the same, regardless of who our mother was.

Moses Nyenswah, my grandfather, was a highly respected town chief. He, too, was a polygamist, with ten wives who bore him multiple children. Revered by his people as a man of valor and compassion, Grandpa was often carried in a hammock on the shoulders of townsmen whenever he traveled because there were no roads and he never walked long distances. After Grandpa's death, all of his children left Panama with their respective mothers to live in nearby villages. But my father decided they all needed to live together in the land of their birth and home of their father. So, he brought all of his younger brothers back to Panama, where he had cultivated the land and expanded the farm. He said that everyone, particularly his siblings, had a stake in maintaining the village.

At the time of my grandfather's death, my father was left alone to care for his mother, Sarah, as well as his brother Robert, who was the youngest of Grandpa's ten living children. When my father married my mother, Sarah was advancing in age and becoming frail. My parents decided to bring my grandmother to live in our home so that our family could take care of her. This was the village tradition.

I was very close to my grandmother. She was warm, doting, and tender. When she moved in with us, I slept in her bed every night and took care of her when she was ill, even though I was a small boy. Grandma died in 1982 from an asthma attack, when I was eight years old. I was saddened by her death and cried myself to sleep because I missed her so much, especially her embrace. She used to hug me so close when I slept with her.

After she died, her body was prepared in our home for burial. The undertaker came to our house and embalmed her in her room. My siblings and I peeked through the door and windows to see what he was doing, but we did not have a clear view from where we stood. All we saw were needles and small bottles. Grandma's body was dressed in her ceremonial best and remained in the house for nearly two weeks as we waited for her family members to arrive from distant places. We waited especially for Uncle Robert, who lived in Monrovia and had to travel the farthest distance. Travel at that time was extremely difficult due to the lack of paved roads and poorly developed road networks. It took days or sometimes weeks to reach Panama from Monrovia.

After what seemed like an eternity, the day finally came when everybody had arrived. A wake was held at our home the night before Grandma Sarah was buried. On the day of her funeral, everyone cried like babies. Grandma was buried in the family graveyard next to her husband's grave. We, the grandchildren, wept even more because both of our grandparents were gone, never to be seen or touched again. My father also cried, though he fought hard to hold back his tears and be the strong man he wanted us to always see. I had never seen my dad cry before.

My mother, Ruth, never went to school and remained completely illiterate her whole life. Yet as a parent she was a strict disciplinarian and instilled in her children the discipline of work. She assigned chores around the house to each child. Everyone had to draw water from the creek and fill a drum. That was our water reservoir. We would heat pots of water for bathing. My mother baked bread in our wood stove, hunted birds, planted rice, and taught us how to weed our rice field. She was a marvelous cook and made sure that we were fed well and always ate our meals together as a family. Our mother loved all her children equally— at least that is what she always said. She always gives us her blessings by putting a pinch of spittle from her mouth on our foreheads, in the Kru tradition. Whenever we travel, she says a prayer, giving us blessings, wishing us good luck, and declaring that we go in peace.

When I was growing up, the polygamous lifestyle was simple to understand and fun for us children. Everybody supported each other. Father rotated his time and affection among his wives, each having one week at a time. Wives and children planted and tilled the farm together. We played and joked together. We ate together out of large pans using our hands. There was no confusion. Each wife knew her place in the polygamous hierarchy. The head wife set the pace, created the schedule, and assigned chores to the others. I thought village life was awesome. We had a lot of fun, despite the simplicity and sometimes deprivation of life.

My siblings and I went to the farm every day to brush the bush, cut palm, hunt with dogs, and swim in the rivers. We walked for hours and carried wood on our heads, then made fires to heat water to bathe. We had to do so much physical work on the farm on weekends that I began to dislike the weekends, longing to be in school when most children longed to be free.

My father only had a second- or third-grade education; yet he thrived because he had street smarts and understood the ways of the world. Although my mother had never entered a schoolroom and was illiterate, she made education a priority for her children. Our village had no dedicated schoolhouse. First- through sixth-grade classrooms were inside the local church building, where we assembled and sat on bare floors; sometimes we sat on loose pieces of wood placed over cinder blocks. Shoeless, we walked about twenty minutes to school, carrying our lunches of cassava, rice, and palm butter prepared by our mother. After school I would carry my books home and change out of my school uniform (green short trousers and white shirt), then walk for an hour to my parents' farm to help with chores. We would return to Panama around five o'clock in the afternoon, carrying water and wood on our heads to make a fire for cooking and to heat water for our parents to bathe.

Every night, my siblings and I would study at the large dining room table. All of our furniture was handmade village furniture. Our house was made of mud, with a zinc roof and whitewashed to make the exterior look like concrete. The bathroom, made of zinc, with a piece of cloth as the door, was a separate structure outside the house. We had electricity in the village. The government-owned electric company provided services at a reasonable cost. The road in front of our house was made of laterite and not paved. We also had electric irons.

My father was prominent in Panama, and many politicians would stop by our house. Despite his educational shortcomings, William Nyenswah was brilliant. He was focused on upward social mobility for himself and his children. Whenever it was expedient, he did what he felt was necessary to promote this mobility. For example, in the past if someone in Liberia did not have an Anglo-Saxon name or come from a prominent family, this was seen as a social impediment. Often, neither a person nor their children could go to school without these privileges, or if they did, the school was likely substandard. Realizing this, William

Nyenswah changed his name to William Moses—his father's first name—thus putting himself in a different social tier.

Americo-Liberians were descendants of freed slaves who came from America and settled in various parts of Liberia, usually around the sea or riverbanks. Reverend Moses, as people referred to my father, adopted the mannerisms of the Americo-Liberians he was striving to emulate. He assumed their way of doing business. He joined the Master Masons and United Brothers Fellowship fraternities and rose to the level of district superintendent in Sinoe. Not only did my father meet President Tolbert when he visited Sinoe to open the Agricultural Camp, but my dad also met Charles Taylor in 1991 and 1992, long before he became president of Liberia in 1997. The Moses home in Panama was graced with the presence of the rich, famous, and infamous. The bishop of the United Methodist Church in Liberia, Rev. Dr. Arthur Flomo Kulah, was also one of our many guests.

Despite changing his last name temporarily—for he reverted to his original name years later—my father gave his children his father's last name, Nyenswah. He strongly believed that the name would become a household name in Liberia someday. He believed that this recognition would come through one of his sons. In his mind, I was the one designated to bring this family name to national prominence. He said he loved all his children equally, but he saw something special in me from birth. Every time we would meet as a family, he would tell us that he was not leaving us houses when he died. He would not amass a fortune to bequeath to us. He would say to us: "If I give you an education, you can build mansions." To me my father also said: "You will be a Joseph of the family. You will save your community. You will save Sinoe County. And one day you will save the Republic of Liberia." This he believed until the day he died. And so, for as long as I can remember, this was imprinted in my mind, in my consciousness. I often wondered why the conviction—why did this man have such confidence in me and my future? Was he a prophet, a soothsayer, a fortune teller, a psychic, or whatever else one might call him? I have thought about this long and hard until I came to the conclusion that my father had a God-given prophecy.

My father had a friendship with Rev. Hamilton C. Russ III and his wife, Nellie. Everyone in the neighborhood, both adults and children, called her Godma. Reverend Russ was the pastor of the First United Methodist Church in Greenville, the capital of Sinoe County, 10 kilometers from Panama by automobile. The reverend was considered very wealthy, civilized, educated, and elite. He was Americo-Liberian, a descendant of freed American slaves who returned to Africa and settled in Liberia.

Often, villagers would send their children to live in Americo-Liberian households, which they believed would provide the educational and future economic opportunities necessary for a better life. The children would be sent to school, which was not usually the best quality, in exchange for services and chores that would otherwise be performed by household help.

Because the public school in our village only went from first through sixth grade, when I was fourteen my parents began negotiating with Reverend Russ to have me live with him in Greenville, in what was known as the Po River Community, so I could continue my education. The negotiations took about a year. Reverend Russ passed away during that time, but my father continued the discussions with Nellie, who agreed that I could live with her. In 1988, I went from our close-knit family to board with the Russ family in Greenville.

I was expected to do chores that I had never done in my life, despite my experience with all the physical labor on my parents' farm. Some of my siblings had gone to other households where the manual labor was too much to bear, which caused them to run back to our parents, forfeiting a primary education for the comfort and love of living with their own family. Many village children finished sixth grade, got married early, and started having children while still very young and inexperienced.

There were other foster children living with the Russ family. Some were not related to the Russes, but others were part of their extended family. It was common in those days for family members of significant means to foster children of family members with lesser means. The Russes' biological children slept in separate rooms in the main house, which was called Russ Palace. In my eyes, it was quite a large structure: a two-story building made of concrete bricks and roofed with zinc—very different from the houses in my village. I slept in the utility house, or "boys' quarters," along with James Harris and Kent Railey, relatives of the Russes who were, like me, servants for the sake of their education.

The Russes had a very large garden, and a herd of animals, all enclosed within a wooden fence. Taking care of the pigs, goats, and cows became one of my responsibilities. I had to get up at five o'clock in the morning to feed the pigs and goats and take the cows to the field before the school day began. After school I brought the animals back into the enclosure to feed them again. I swept the yard of the debris that had fallen from the large plum trees that shaded the garden. I would later learn that what are known as mangoes in other countries are considered plums in Liberia.

Coming from a village where life was simple and relatively free—where I knew I was loved by my parents and siblings and where we had so much fun and laughter every day—I felt that the new life that my father hoped would better my social status was more like servitude. It was child labor. The workload was unbearable. Never in my village life had I done the things for which I was responsible or expected to do in the Russes' home. I became very angry with my parents for sending me to live with these people. I used to howl in frustration and retreat to the woods where I would cry and spend quiet time alone. Kent often encouraged me to be strong and bear it. He said my life would get better in the end. Even though I listened to him, I still entertained the thought of running away and going back to the home I loved so much. I thought of fleeing just as some of my other siblings had done.

I learned which of the other children could be trusted and which to avoid. Of Reverend Russ's biological children, Cathy was studious and privileged, yet kind and approachable—unlike her sister Florence, the only child of Nellie Russ. Cathy treated me as a brother and made living with her family tolerable. But Florence was spoiled. She was tough and unfriendly. We were servants in her eyes, having to cater to her every need. Of all the children in the house, she was the only one allowed to bring her friends over. The rest of us, including Cathy, were not allowed to bring a soul into the yard, let alone into the house.

Kent was exceptionally gracious. He genuinely cared about my well-being. His parents provided food for the Russes' animals and also lived in Greenville. He would invite me into his parents' home to eat every time we went to pick up food for the animals. Kent, James, and I slept together in one room in the boys' quarters. At night we would cook food in an isolated area at the back of the house. We would have been in big trouble if Mrs. Russ had found out. We would catch crabs and cook them under the moonlight as we watched the stars. The stars shone so bright against the midnight sky, and it reminded me of nights in my village when our whole family would sit around the kitchen outside together, watching the stars and eating delicious food.

The Russes' home was a two-story, two-family house that stood on four acres of very fertile land that was fenced in to accommodate and protect their animals. The property included one hundred and fifty acres of undeveloped land, surrounded by a lagoon on one side, with the ocean nearby. The Russes lived on the ground level, or first story as we called it, and rented the second story to Ms. Jugbeh Harris and Mr. Divine Aggor, a manager of Shell Oil Company, who was from the Volta Region, Republic of Ghana. From the second floor, one could see the sea. It was a clear, stunning vista. Jugbeh was a Kru woman, who often gave Kent and me food in exchange for doing handy work and odd jobs, much to the displeasure of Mrs. Russ, so we would hide behind the utility house, under the coconut and plum (mango) trees, which provided shade like a canopy.

Being near the sea was comforting because I was accustomed to being near the water in Panama. The Russes' property was also adjacent to Po River, where we set traps to catch crabs, steaming or roasting them on the fire we made at night. As servants, we were only given one meal a day, so catching crabs provided us with a second meal that we desperately needed. We would also go swimming in the river, which was something I commonly did in Panama. One day Mrs. Russ discovered that I had been swimming in the river. She became terribly angry and called her brother, who lived nearby. She told him to beat me with his saw. He violently struck me as she yelled, "I don't want your country, native parents to say I killed you or drowned you in the river!" I did not understand why swimming would provoke such a negative reaction. Thereafter, Mrs. Russ would regularly summon her brother to beat me and the other foster children with the carpenter's saw for what I considered minor infractions. Sometimes he would beat me with a stick called the "yellow hull," which is a very straight sticklike plant that is yellow with green leaves. People used this rod to beat their servants because of its rigidity, strength, and durability. Mrs. Russ kept her yellow hull locked in her room and would often use it to thrash us. Most of the time I had no idea what I had done to deserve a beating. At times like this, I longed for my home in the village and my parents, friends, and siblings, all of whom I missed beyond measure.

In 1989, the civil war started in Liberia. Most of the children at the Russ' home returned to live with their parents, which left me there alone. Not only did I feel isolated, but I was burdened with more work because I had to take up all of their chores. I was desperately seeking a way out of this hellhole. Then, I found out that my sister Agnes was living with her boyfriend in nearby Greenville. In anguish, I reached out to her to rescue me. Without hesitation, Agnes arranged for me to live with them.

The day I left, I became ill with a headache, fever, and malaria. Mrs. Russ refused to take me to the hospital, though I pleaded with her through tears and suffering. My pain turned into anger. I decided to leave. I would fend for myself, come what may. I built up my courage and walked up to Mrs. Russ in her living room.

"I am leaving your house," I said. "Thank you for all you've done for me to go to school."

"You can leave," she replied. "You country children don't like to be disciplined."

Her daughter Florence stood by her, shouting, "Let him go, Ma! Stupid country, native children."

With tears rolling down my face, I walked out of the living room door, out of the house, and never looked back.

I will always remember that day. That was the day I set myself free.

Unsafe Rituals, Burial Practices, and International Spread

In April and most of May 2014, the epidemic seemed to be abating. Lofa County remained the epicenter in Liberia, with the highest concentration of new cases and mortalities. At that time, the World Health Organization's Disease Outbreak News reported about the Ebola situation in West Africa, saying that there were "no new confirmed cases in Liberia" or described the situation as "stable."[1]

At the beginning of the second phase of the outbreak (May–July 2014), for several weeks, new cases appeared to decrease significantly throughout the country.[1] Then a new case was detected in Monrovia, followed by a rapid escalation in reported new cases in the capital by mid-June. The Ministry of Health and Social Welfare (MOHSW) was forced to admit that there would be an onslaught of new Ebola cases and the health system as a whole was ill-prepared to cope with the overload of infections that would follow. We felt as if we had been ambushed and there was nowhere to escape to.[1]

Despite the national slogans plastered and broadcast all over the place, members of traditional societies—particularly those in rural communities, and former rural dwellers now living in Monrovia—continued to engage in unsafe rituals and burial practices. They bathed the dead, dressed the dead, touched the dead in various ways, and exposed their children to the dead and to water used to wash the dead. Some secretly buried the dead without reporting the death to authorities. Whole households and families died after these secret funerals.

Tradition dictates certain rituals be performed by close family members before burial. Even though touching a corpse infected with Ebola or being exposed to body fluids increased the risk of transmission, people simply did not want to forego these burial rituals to save their own lives. There are many traditional beliefs concerning what will happen to the living if these traditions are not practiced. It was a challenge to educate people to make them aware of Ebola's dangers and bring them to an understanding of the possibility of disease and death, especially at a time when many border towns were hard hit by Ebola.

In July, a safe burial team was established because corpses were lying in the streets of Monrovia, increasing the risk of infection to local communities. People were so afraid of dying from Ebola that whenever a member in a household showed any signs or symptoms of the disease, they were isolated or thrown out of the house. Those with the disease in the advanced stage, with no place to go, died in the streets. Those who died in the house were thrown into the streets. With corpses everywhere, the stench from decaying bodies permeated the city. People in communities were afraid to leave their homes. Monrovia's streets had become graveyards.

The government took charge to safely remove corpses from the streets and from people's homes by creating a Dead Body Management (DBM) team, consisting predominantly of environmental health workers primarily from within MOHSW. Young community volunteers also became part of the team. The DBM team was trained by WHO infection prevention and control (IPC) specialists from Geneva and WHO Africa Region. The goal was to promote safety of the team in handling infected corpses. Mark Y. Korvayan, an environmental health technician at MOHSW, was appointed head of DBM. Mark E. Nyenti, Jah Lawrence Hill, Kiyee Friday, Aloysius J. Cooper, and others constituted the team of body carriers.

There were no designated trucks to move corpses off the street, and nobody in town would rent us their trucks, so I met with MOHSW Procurement Manager Jacob Wapoe, Deputy Minister of Administration Honorable Matthew T. K. Flomo, and Comptroller Toagoe Karzon to convince them to buy two trucks for the team. We purchased the trucks from a Chinese garage near the Nigerian Embassy on Tubman Boulevard in Congo Town.

Dressed in personal protective equipment, DBM removed truckloads of dead bodies from the streets. The question remained: where would we bury the bodies? Community resistance to burial of Ebola-infested bodies in their communities was the order of the day. Many who lived in communities near rivers, creeks, and other bodies of water believed that burying the body of one who had died of Ebola would contaminate the soil and Ebola would be transmitted to community waters. Consequently, dead bodies began to pile up in the trucks.

The search for a suitable burial ground took me and the burial team to Kissi Camp, near a place called Kpeh-kpeh Town, in Johnsonville, a township about thirty miles outside of Monrovia. Here again, there was resistance, resulting in three days of contention between security forces and community dwellers, who claimed the land was private property and worried that their health would be seriously compromised by the corpses.

I sought the advice of the minister of internal affairs, Hon. Morris Dukuly, who cochaired the Presidential Task Force on Ebola. He assured me that his department had negotiated for and purchased the land in Johnsonville to be used as a burial ground for these bodies. So, in fact, the government owned the land. After the clearance was received and the land secured, burial was delayed because the first bulldozer taken to the site got stuck in the mud. It was the rainy season. Though we spent hours trying to remove the truck from the mud, we could not. The mud was like slippery clay. We hired another bulldozer, capable of digging through the mud. In the meantime, I asked MOHSW authorities to immediately purchase machetes, hooks, diggers, and shovels so we could do manual excavation to begin the burial in a mass grave. At one point, I was told there were forty-five bodies to be buried, then sixty-five, then the number rose to an unspecified number, which far exceeded what I thought we had. I personally led the team to remove truckloads of corpses from the ELWA Ebola treatment unit (ETU) (specifically, ELWA 3-MSF) and buried them in Johnsonville township.

We made mistakes. Some of the corpses were buried in wetlands. These corpses were left in a hole that was not properly excavated; when it rained that night, some of the bodies were seen floating in the water on the ground the next morning. In the torrential rain, the area had flooded so badly, it looked like a river overflowing. Although we had on rain boots, the water came over some of our boots. We knew then that we had to get out of that place. Residents in Johnsonville saw dead bodies floating in the streets, and someone called the press. In what seemed like a split second, journalists were all over the place, taking pictures and wanting to talk to us. We managed to escape without being interviewed. The next morning, local newspapers carried the story. One headline read: "Ebola Corpses Dumped in Wetlands." National and international news outlets picked up the story. It was an embarrassing moment for the burial team, for me in particular, and for the MOHSW. We simply were not prepared for this situation.

Corpses continued to accumulate on the streets. In Monrovia, we had one official burial team, with only six men. The workload was overwhelming and, as a result, there was a backlog in collecting corpses. People were dying in record numbers, their bodies thrown out on the streets. It was devastating to see people watching their loved ones being put into body bags.

As people came to the ELWA ETU and died, they needed to be buried quickly to make space to admit other patients for urgent care and treatment. Maybe, just maybe, some would survive. As soon as we got the two assigned trucks, I led the DBM team to the ELWA ETU and picked up a plethora of corpses.

Meanwhile, on the other side of town, about thirty miles away, in the densely populated district of Clara Town, Ebola victims were left to lie on the street for sometimes four days, in seventy-eight-degree heat, when no one would dare to take them to the hospital, creating an intolerable stench. This was concerning because Clara Town is known to exist under extremely poor sanitary conditions, often with no toilet facilities in the houses, a likely death trap during the epidemic. Whenever community residents fell ill and sought help from other community members, often the community members ran for their lives. No hospital beds or ETUs were available in Clara Town or adjacent areas at this stage.

On July 23, a disgruntled, grieving relative of an Ebola victim came to the ministry pretending to be a visitor and set fire to the main conference room on the fourth floor of the MOHSW building, forcing staff members to evacuate.

The situation prompted President Ellen Johnson Sirleaf and her government to make a strong policy decision on cremation. By mid-August, the government announced that it would "consider cremating" the corpses of those who had died from EVD. The directive came from the president to me as the incident manager, that all Ebola victims in Liberia should be cremated to curtail the spread of infection from highly contagious corpses and prevent the unsightly accumulation of corpses in the streets.

Boye's Town, on the Roberts International Airport Highway, was chosen and established as the cremation site. Citizens and traditional leaders protested. The idea of cremation induced deep fear in traditional societies; people believed they would go straight to hell if cremated. Cremating the dead had never been a part of the Liberian culture.

Under heavy military escort, I accompanied the burial team to the makeshift crematory in Boye's Town. Two mini trucks carrying Ebola-infected corpses to the crematory site were guarded on each side by a heavily armed platoon of soldiers from the Liberian Army and officers from the Liberia National Police Support Unit (PSU), which functions as a riot squad. Each corpse lay in a secured body bag, accompanied by a corresponding plywood peg bearing the deceased's name, age, and date of death.

Bodies shrouded by a body bag were left in piles at the cremation site, awaiting the actual cremation ceremony. This would have never been achieved without the government's deployment of security forces at the site around the clock.

In response to the president's directive, people stopped taking sick relatives to the ETU, fearing that they would be cremated. Instead, they hid the sick and secretly buried the dead; in the process, they were infected themselves, thereby dramatically increasing the Ebola case load and fatality rates in Liberia.

On July 20, Patrick Sawyer traveled from Liberia to Lagos, Nigeria, on a Nigerian airline. Sawyer, a naturalized American citizen who was born in Liberia, was working as a consultant with the Ministry of Finance and Development Planning. Upon arrival at Murtala Muhammed International Airport in Lagos, Sawyer appeared ill, exhibiting what authorities believed were signs and symptoms of Ebola. The Nigerian airport authorities isolated him immediately and transported him to the First Consultant Hospital, a nearby private hospital on Lagos Island's Obalende neighborhood,[2,3] where his condition worsened. While rendering care, several of the medical staff, including Dr. Ameyo Stella Adadevoh, the doctor who admitted him, were exposed to his bodily fluids. Sawyer was tested and confirmed positive for Ebola. He died shortly thereafter, having started a secondary outbreak. Dr. Adadevoh subsequently died on August 19, 2014, as did other Nigerians.[4,5,6] The Nigerian team of public health professionals rapidly initiated a contact tracing team in Lagos to track all those who may have been in proximity to Sawyer during his travels and those in contact with infected hospital staff. To ensure that no contact got away, contact tracing was extended to other parts of Nigeria, to which some contacts were suspected of traveling. As a result, Ebola was rapidly contained in Nigeria and the case fatality rate kept to a minimum. Dr. Adadevoh was credited with preventing a massive spread of Ebola in Nigeria by insisting Patrick Sawyer be quarantined and refusing to release him, despite being pressured—even threatened—by Liberian government officials who wanted him released to attend a conference.[7,8]

This was the first time that Ebola had transcended the borders of the three affected Mano River countries, since its emergence in Guinea in December 2013. It was no longer an "exotic disease" limited to three countries in West Africa. Now at last, western countries began to see the West African Ebola epidemic as a public health emergency. Only then did they take heed of President Sirleaf's desperate plea for help to save the lives of the people of Liberia.

Nigeria immediately halted all air transport to and from Liberia. Considering that Nigerian airlines provided most of the air transport in the West African region, this decision became a tremendous inconvenience for people who had to travel out of Liberia, as other airlines also limited travel to and from that country. According to CDC Director Tom Frieden, "Ebola is worsening in West Africa," announcing the level 3 advisory—its strongest level—against travel to Liberia, Guinea, and Sierra Leone. Frieden said the CDC was sending fifty additional staff to West Africa to advise countries on controlling the disease, adding, "It's the largest, most complex (Ebola) outbreak that we know of in history."[9] When the team got on the ground, I presented them with a strategy that we had developed on every aspect of the response, including building treatment units, the amount of bed space needed to treat patients, personal protective equipment (PPE) needs, and financial plans.

It was discovered that Sawyer may have already known he had Ebola. His sister had died of Ebola a few weeks earlier in Liberia, and he had been in close contact with her during her illness, as well as with her corpse.[10,11,12] In fact, Patrick's sister was treated at Saint Joseph's Catholic Hospital, where the administrator and nurses contracted the virus.

On August 1, the president of Guinea hosted a meeting with the presidents of Liberia and Sierra Leone in Conakry to address this regional public health emergency. Dr. Margaret Chan, WHO director-general at the time, was present.[13] She encouraged the leaders to take full responsibility and act definitively. She assured them that WHO would provide technical guidance and increased material support.

Dr. Chan also outlined potential outcomes of a prolonged outbreak and the risk of global seclusion, if certain restrictive measures were not imposed on border crossings and commercial activities.[13] Following the meeting, the presidents issued a joint declaration to use the military and police to isolate the cross-border areas. Provisions for necessary support to the population in these areas was included in the declaration.

If the declaration could not get the attention of the international community, infected foreigners could. On July 23, two American missionaries were diagnosed with EVD. Dr. Kent Brantley, a physician, and Nancy Writebol, a nurse, had been working for Samaritan's Purse at ELWA's ETU.[14,15,16] They had been stationed in Liberia prior to the onset on the epidemic.[17] The fact that they were infected raised the alarm in the United States of the situation in Liberia. Much effort was made by the Americans to save the lives of these two citizens. At the beginning of August, the two missionaries were evacuated by private air ambulance from Liberia to the CDC in Atlanta, Georgia. Both would recover and be discharged from CDC facilities on August 21.[18]

A Liberian hygienist, also employed at ELWA's ETU, died on July 27 after contracting EVD. International media attention heightened when the experimental drug ZMapp (based on humanized monoclonal antibodies to Ebola virus) was brought to Liberia by Samaritan's Purse for the sole purpose of treating its American employees. While the Americans were evacuated to the United States by air ambulance, several Liberian physicians in the ETU became infected with the Ebola virus; one of whom was Dr. Samuel Brisbane, the head of the Internal Medicine Department at the John F. Kennedy Medical Center in Monrovia.

The dramatic evacuation of the two Americans prompted President Sirleaf to request, on humanitarian grounds, the same drug for Liberian citizens. There was further public outcry after the evacuation. People expressed more anger and distrust of the government and of the Americans, who seemed to not care whether Liberians lived or die. The public was incensed that the Liberian hygienist was a mere footnote, while the Americans got the expensive preferential treatment. The fact that people were dying in other settings outside of ETUs, with no hope in sight, further compounded the problem.

On August 5, the Brothers Hospitallers of Saint John of God, an international Catholic order that provides health and social services around the world, confirmed that Spaniard Brother Miguel Pajares had been infected after volunteering in Liberia. The Spanish military assisted with his transfer on August 6. Authorities stated he would be treated in the Carlos III Hospital in Madrid. This attracted controversy, amid questions as to the authorities' ability to guarantee no risk of transmission. Brother Pajares died from the virus on August 12.[19]

By August, the epidemic had reached close to 2,000 cases; 80 cases were being reported each day, sometimes up to 600 a week in Liberia alone.[20] The social and economic fabric of the country was fast eroding.[21,22] The EVD outbreak had strained government finances, increased national deficits, and resulted in drastic shortfalls in domestic revenue. These substantial impacts would ripple beyond the borders of the most affected countries and carry an estimated regional economic cost of US$500,000 to $6.2 billion, indicating the inextricable linkages between health system resilience, socioeconomic development and growth, and global security.[21,22] This created an unprecedented impetus to address critical health system vulnerabilities to build resilience against future shocks, in tandem with broader multisector reconstruction and recovery.[23]

In July, only WHO, MSF, and USAID were providing technical and financial support to the MOHSW. MSF was the lone international agency supporting the government in terms of advocacy and calling on the international community to support the response effort. WHO's response was handicapped due to the lack of adequate support from member states. I could sense the frustration from the WHO country representative, Dr. Nestor Ndayimirije, and witnessed the tension in the room between and among the international responders. MSF was very vocal and did not hesitate to express how extremely frustrated they were with the slow pace of commitment of both financial and technical resources from the international community. The international response to the Ebola outbreak was late. Many of those who came to aid us would not arrive until late September and October, by which time we Liberians had figured out that if the world didn't respond to President Sirleaf's plea for financial, technical, and logistical assistance, we had to find a way to save ourselves.

Much to our chagrin, international donations were not forthcoming. As cases multiplied and fatality rates soared, the government of Liberia and its people recognized that the international community was not coming to our aid. Foreign donor countries, international aid agencies, and private foundations failed to acknowledge that the Ebola outbreak constituted a major public health and humanitarian crisis, and it was not restricted to a local health sector problem. United Nations officials seemed not to appreciate that the Ebola epidemic presented safety hazards and security risks, even though there were established UN structures in Liberia, with the WHO leading the response, along with the MOHSW.

In the midst of the epidemic, WHO was having its own internal crisis. During the outbreak, the WHO Liberia Country Office changed its country representative three times.

Dr. Nestor Ndayimirije, who had been country representative for several years, was suddenly recalled to WHO's Africa Region headquarters in Brazzaville, Congo, temporarily replaced by Peter Graff. After several months, Dr. Alex Gasasira, who had come from an external WHO post to provide technical assistance to Liberia's Ebola response, would become country representative. At the Ministry of Health, we believed these changes were a result of challenging demands in an unprecedented epidemic. We also believed that politics within the collective international community may have played a role in Dr. Ndayimirije's recall from his post. Minister of Health Gwenigale felt it necessary to come to Dr. Ndayimirije's defense when he was being forcefully criticized by prominent officials of international institutions on the ground. Gwenigale had worked closely with his WHO colleague and trusted his advice unequivocally. He was not prepared to allow his professional integrity to be destroyed.

On July 27, Liberia closed most of its border crossings. Schools were closed on July 30. About a week later, on August 4, the US ambassador to Liberia, Deborah Malac, declared a disaster. On August 6, on national television, President Sirleaf declared a state of emergency and imposed a nationwide dusk-to-dawn curfew.[24] WHO then convened an "Emergency Committee to assess the Ebola situation under the provisions in the International Health Regulations."[25] In a meeting on August 8, the committee agreed that "the Ebola outbreaks constituted a public health emergency of international concern." The following day, Director-General Chan declared the same.[25] On August 8, the World Health Organization called Ebola in West Africa a public health emergency of international concern (PHEIC).[20] WHO defines a PHEIC as "an extraordinary event that may constitute a public health risk to other countries through international spread of disease and may require an international coordinated response." The purpose for the declaration of a PHEIC is to focus international attention on acute public health risks that "require coordinated mobilization of extraordinary resources by the international community" for prevention and response."[26] With this announcement, the world became aware that Ebola was no longer geographically confined to three West African countries. It had traveled across international boundaries and could spread to any corner of the globe at any time. Rich and poor were equally vulnerable. Patrick Sawyer had changed the global perception of Ebola transmission when he brought Ebola to Nigeria.

WHO's declaration included a recommendation that countries should refrain from putting travel restrictions that could affect trade and isolate Guinea, Liberia, and Sierra Leone.[27,28,29] However, despite the PHEIC declaration and recommendation to halt travel restrictions, by the end of August almost every country in the world would have implemented some type of mandatory restrictions on international travel, specifically restrictions against Guineans, Liberians, and Sierra Leoneans. In most instances, entry was denied based on nationality or travel history, resulting in suspension of air travel and visa restrictions, among other actions. As the outbreak spread, many countries also closed their borders to most international travelers, especially from West Africa, an unprecedented situation.

Despite the restrictions, in mid-September, a Liberian national, Thomas Eric Duncan, would travel by air to the United States, where he presented with symptoms of Ebola. Staff at the Texas hospital where he initially appeared seeking treatment apparently were not aware of the signs and symptoms of Ebola and therefore did not appropriately treat Duncan, nor did they protect themselves with personal protective equipment. Several nurses became infected after exposure to his blood and bodily fluids. Duncan would later be given the experimental drug brincidofovir on October 4, but he died shortly thereafter, becoming the first diagnosed Ebola death in the United States.[30,31,32] The infected nurses were flown to the National Institutes of Health (NIH) in Bethesda, Maryland, where they received supportive treatment and survived.[30,31,32]

With Ebola unexpectedly in America, more people became aware that the West African Ebola epidemic posed a global public health threat. Global health security quickly became the priority for Western governments. Meanwhile, in Monrovia, international organizations were evacuating their international staff, leaving Liberian staff behind to die. Foreign embassies in Monrovia, including the United States Embassy, evacuated nonessential staff and their families. Many Liberians who had the financial means or had families in Europe or America, left the country, as did expatriates in various industries.

Nine months had passed since the start of the outbreak before WHO proclaimed it a "public health emergency of international concern." The delay of the declaration, I believe, resulted in the loss of innocent lives that could have been saved. As a public health expert sounding the warning in Liberia in the initial stages of the outbreak, I felt the slow pace of the international response was disingenuous! Never again should this happen in the world.

CHAPTER 4

A Refugee in Côte d'Ivoire

On August 26, Dr. Tom Frieden, then director of the US Centers for Disease Control and Prevention (CDC), arrived in Liberia to assess the Ebola outbreak. He called the "overwhelming" situation "a crisis." From Monrovia, opposition politicians accused the government of doing little or nothing to halt the outbreak. Frieden told National Public Radio (NPR), "They need a lot of help from the world. . . . The real question is how much worse will it get? How many more people will be infected and how much more risk to the world will there be?" Frieden referenced the prolonged civil war that killed 250,000 people, acknowledging that Liberia had suffered even before Ebola struck. "Liberia has been through so much in the last fifteen or twenty years," Frieden said. "This is really almost re-traumatizing people here."[1]

By September 23, the *New York Times* reported, quoting the CDC projections, that "Ebola cases could reach 1.4 million cases in just four months."[2] In another news report, ABC News put it like this: "without the proper intervention, the Ebola outbreak could reach 1.4 million cases by the end of January, according to new estimates from the U.S. Centers for Disease Control and Prevention."[3] As the lead person of the government's response, I was consulted about the mathematical modeling prior to the public announcement. The goal was for me to brief President Ellen Johnson Sirleaf of the austere future predictions— and to prepare her for an uphill battle.

When the First Liberian Civil War began, in 1989, I was fifteen years old and living at the Russes' home. After I decided to leave my life of enslavement under Mrs. Russ, as I perceived it, I went to Greenville, where I lived for several months with my elder sister, Agnes; her boyfriend; and my younger sister, Sharon. I sold cold water in the mornings to earn an income and help with expenses, and I went to school in the afternoons. Even though I assisted with chores, it was a joy not to work like a servant, as I had for Mrs. Russ. I was with my beloved sisters.

The civil war was started by Charles Taylor, the former director of the General Services Agency in President Samuel K. Doe's government. While on official travel duties to the United States, Taylor was accused of embezzlement. Charges were brought against him and a formal request was made to the US government for his extradition. He was arrested in Boston, Massachusetts, and jailed in a maximum security prison from which he escaped and left the United States. It was said he fled to Mexico initially, then to Ghana and subsequently to Libya, where his friend Muammar Gaddafi was president. There, he trained as a mercenary and recruited other mercenaries—from Libya, Burkina Faso, and Gambia—who joined him in invading Liberia in December 1989. Other Liberian rebels joined forces with Taylor in a vicious attempt to oust President Doe. The invasion began in Bhutuo, Nimba County, and moved into the country's numerous rural, densely forested counties in 1990. That is when it reached Sinoe County.

As the war intensified, I decided to return home to my village in Panama to reunite with my family. Following the closure of all schools, the situation quickly worsened. My family became internally displaced— forced to leave our homes but remaining in our country—as were many others in the villages and towns in Sinoe County. We witnessed people being massacred. The rebel fighters killed civilians indiscriminately, looted and burned down many houses, and raped and enslaved young girls. Young boys—the same age as my brothers and me—were conscripted into the rebel factions. It was terrifying!

My father's adaptive behavior led him to the forests of Sinoe, where we made a farm, as a means of growing food to feed our family. He, my brothers, and I mined artisanal gold. Digging gold became my way of life from 1991 to 1993. There was no law and order. We were living in the bush, in thick forests, working for rebels and warlords. The rebels bought our gold and paid us much less than the gold was worth, though it was enough to buy additional food, which we could not grow. We also exchanged gold for rice, salt, and other food. These rebels were fearless, and in order to do business with them we, too, became fearless. If we were to survive the war, that was the only way.

Sinoe County was one of the richest areas for gold mining in Liberia. We used unconventional tools: cutlasses, shovels, and pieces of old rugs to catch the gold and other items. Our days began at six o'clock in the morning, and we worked until seven o'clock in the evening. Mining gold was hard, manual labor. We had no choice but to do it. The rebels and soldiers would beat us mercilessly and put us in prison if we did not give them a sizable percentage of our earnings. They looted villages and terrorized people. Some chose to join the rebels for the free food and guaranteed protection. My interactions with the rebels were very limited.

The Liberian Peace Council (LPC) was one of the rebel factions headed by ex-warlord Dr. George Boley, who had been the minister of education under President Doe. Boley's rebel forces seized the city of Greenville, in Sinoe County, from Charles Taylor's rebel forces (the National Patriotic Front) and occupied the city for an extended period of time. At some point after this occupation but during the civil crisis, George Boley left Liberia for the United States. In March 2012, US Immigration and Customs Enforcement deported him from the United States to Liberia, for allegedly committing human rights abuses during the Liberian civil war. This was "the first-ever removal under the

Child Soldiers Accountability Act."[4] Back in Liberia, he ran for political office and was elected district representative for Grand Gedeh County in 2017.

The Nyenswahs had stayed put during the early years of the conflict because the rebels led by Charles Taylor were not as brutal to the Kru people in Sinoe. Over time, however, ethnic conflict escalated. Rumors led to actual rifts that intensified quickly and turned into a tribal and regional conflict. The Gio, part of the mountain-dwelling Dan tribe, began pursuing the Sapo-speaking people, whom they considered a part of Doe's ethnic group, the Krahns. The Krahns constitute a part of the seafaring Kru tribe. To defend themselves, the Sapo began spreading stories that the Krus were leading the Gio on a campaign to exterminate the Sapos. This of course was untrue. There is a long-standing relationship, between the Kru and Sapo people, dating back to the founding of Liberia. My uncle Peter was married to a Sapo woman and in Greenville I went to school with many Sapo friends. We did not know or recognize the difference until the civil war. Nonetheless, these rumors led to increased fighting near our village that threatened lives and property, forcing distressed villagers to leave their homes.

As bloodshed intensified between Kru and Sapo tribal leadership, in October 1993 we decided to leave Sinoe County. George Boley's rebels had entered the city with heavy gunfire. I ran through the village to my parents. My maternal grandmother, Sarah Peters, was blind as a result of glaucoma. We could not leave her alone. She needed to be guided. My father, mother, grandmother, sixteen siblings, and I began walking from Sinoe to the neighboring Grand Kru County on footpaths that took us from village to village, town to town. We were mentally exhausted, living with uncertainty about our future. I carried my grandmother on my back for most of the journey. At nineteen years old, I was strong, and I knew that transporting her on my back was the fastest way for us to move through the bush. I loved my grandma. As a boy, I spent most of my time with her. I would cook food with her. I slept in her bed, cuddled in her arms, and was rocked to sleep many nights by her. For me, carrying her on my back was a duty and a privilege. As we walked through the bush, we reminisced about our village life and talked about how things had suddenly changed. She gave me her blessings for being a capable and devoted grandson. I will always remember her compassionate words and all her blessings. I firmly believe they carry me through every day of my life, no matter what challenges I face.

Never during my childhood had this mass exodus from our native country been foretold. Our life in Panama was all forests and tall, green grass and a big family with sixteen children. We started each day with prayers and Bible verses. At Christmastime we sang carols, and the sound of our voices would resonate throughout our home. Now that this war had reached Sinoe County, our lives were disrupted, our village destroyed, and we were forced to roam in places unknown. We obtained the title of *internally displaced* during our roaming and became *refugees* when we crossed over into the Ivory Coast. We were all devastated by our newly evolving status, both the young and the old.

Being refugees was a difficult thing for our parents, who had been living a stable life in their village. Now they, their children, and their elders had moved into the bush. There was no safe drinking water, food, or shelter. We had no clue where we would end up. We were constantly at risk of contracting diseases, suffering diarrhea from drinking polluted water, and being malnourished due to lack of food. We watched people die from communicable diseases. Sanitation was a major issue, as we relieved ourselves along the walking path. We were frightened of dying in the forest and rotting there. It was a punishing time for us as children, because suddenly we had to grow up fast. We lived in fear and depended on our parents to keep us safe, though they themselves were not certain how they could protect us, their precious children, or even themselves. One thing was clear: none of us wanted to join any rebel group.

Our family traveled together through the bush to avoid being found by rebel soldiers, who stuck to the road. We inched our way along footpaths, some of which had been overgrown by weeds and other plants, using our cutlasses to clear our way. We traveled from Kpanyan District, Panama, through Dugbe River Districts, spending weeks, sometimes months in towns and villages, while always hoping to go back to Panama soon. That hope faded, after we spent about three months in Seaton Town, four months in Sayoa, and six months in Nhamkankop. Then we ended up on the beaches in Grand Kru, where we stayed in Sobo Town, then Pattay Town, for longer than expected. It was difficult to find food, so we lived primarily on cassava roots and boiled water from the Atlantic Ocean, which we also used to extract salt to season our food.

In Grand Kru, we lived on the beach for a month. Our father, being an elder in full connection (ministers formally prepared for "ministry of the Word, Sacrament, and Order"; they are also ordained) in the Methodist Church, was recognized by one of the Methodist elders of the Sobo group, who arranged accommodations for us. Our family was divided into several small groups and given shelter in various houses in different locations. There were no toilets in these houses, so we had to defecate and urinate on the beach or in the sea. Many of the Sobo people in Grand Kru were fishermen, and they taught us a lot. We learned how to cast fishing nets early in the morning and haul them in in the evening, adding bait cannons to catch fish for our entire family. Although we were scattered among multiple houses with strangers, we were able to meet as a family some evenings. As a young man, I bore the greatest burden of providing for my family and picked up whatever jobs were available. I was a gold digger at one time, traded palm oil occasionally, and often went to sea to catch fish, either to sell or for my family to eat. We also collected saltwater from the ocean, boiling large quantities of it until the water evaporated. We would then extract the salt to sell. Our father was vehemently against the rebel factions and wanted us to play no part in their activities, so we made do with what we could.

Our life on the beach was cut short when the rebels moved into Grand Kru. As they advanced closer, our family began walking again. Crossing the war zone was both physically and emotionally grueling. As we trekked, we witnessed soldiers slaughtering people along the roadside. We watched soldiers killing women and children, as well as grown men. Dead bodies washed ashore on the beaches around Pattay

Town, Sobo Town, Nifu Town, Sobobo, and Sasstown, all the way up to Grandcess. Young boys and sometimes girls were regularly conscripted as child soldiers. Our family attempted to forestall this tragedy by drawing up a plan. The adults would hide the children whenever they felt a threat, or the older youth would put our mothers on our backs and pretend that they were sick whenever we encountered soldiers. Despite these precautionary measures, on one occasion my brothers Swen, Abraham, Wleh, and I were captured by rebels and taken to Nifu Town. They gave us guns and instructed us to man a checkpoint. When they fell asleep, we escaped and returned to our family.

It took another month to walk from Grand Kru to Pleebo in Maryland County. To purchase food and other necessities, we bought palm oil from Decoris Oil Palm Company in Pleebo Sodokan district, to sell in the Ivory Coast because the selling price there was much higher than in Pleebo. After each purchase, we transferred the oil into five-gallon containers and my brother Swen and I each transported five of these containers by foot, in wheelbarrows, from Pleebo to the Cavalla River crossing, a distance of 103 miles. The Cavalla River creates a boundary between Liberia and the Ivory Coast. It took us a full twenty-four hours to walk with our loaded wheelbarrows, often making multiple rest stops in the scorching heat. Sometimes we perspired so profusely that we had to take off our shirts to wring out the sweat and hang them to dry, as we looked for shaded areas near villages on the road, to rest and find food. Usually, after arrival at the river crossing, we had to sleep by the river bank before crossing the next morning. In the morning, we boarded large commercial cargo / passenger canoes and crossed the border into Côte d'Ivoire. We use the names Ivory Coast (English) and Côte d'Ivoire (French) interchangeably. After docking we had to walk about an hour to Gozon, the border town, where we sold our oil. Making these trips was long and difficult. We traded oil in this way once a week for many months, making four round trips a month. In Gozon, we used the money we earned from our sales to buy food and other supplies to take back home to our family in Pleboo. The prices and quality of goods were much better in the Ivory Coast than in Liberia.

We were settling down quite well in Pleebo until the rebels came to Maryland County in early 1994, forcing the Nyenswah clan to trek to the Cavalla River crossing to board passenger canoes to the Ivory Coast. After the long walk and having to carry my grandmother on my back most of the way, relieved for short breaks by one of my brothers, we had to wait three full days before we could cross. The passenger canoes could only carry six or seven people and their belongings, and there was a huge crowd of multiple families also waiting to cross. Due to our large family size, we had to travel in several cramped canoes. On the way, we saw other boats capsize and watched as many women and their little children drowned. People were rushing to board the boats because of the sound of gunfire everywhere. More gunfire came from the city of Pleebo, the sound reverberating all the way to the crossing point. The rebels had lined the riverbank and were shooting at everything in sight. A man named Nate, also known as Rebel King, a notorious rebel leader, was leading a large group of rebels, mostly teenage boys. They were accusing civilians of harboring opposition rebel groups in their homes and communities. They intended to find them, kill them, and punish those who hid them as brutally as possible, if they chose not to kill them. We were terrified. Hearing that indiscriminate gunfire, we knew we had to leave Liberia. By the grace of God, our entire family made it across the river. When we docked in Côte d'Ivoire, we cried out loud, thanking God as we said goodbye to Liberia.

For weeks, we slept in open fields without proper shelter and survived by cooking and eating roots and weeds that we seasoned with our homemade sea salt. Boiling seawater was the only way to get salt until the United Nations High Commission on Refugees (UNHCR) and the Adventist Development and Relief Agency (ADRA) opened an enormous refugee camp near the village of Gozon. My parents decided we should go to the camp site and take our chances.

When we finally arrived at the Gozon refugee camp, we had been walking for four to five months, when you consider the walk from Sinoe, through Grand Kru, into Maryland County and then to the Cavalla River before crossing over into Ivory Coast. To our dismay, Gozon was a terrible place—much worse than other places we had been in Sinoe and Grand Kru. Our previous visits there to trade oil were limited to the short distance from the river dock to the Gozon market. The camp hosted over 10,000 people. There was no housing. There were no toilets. There was, at first, no food.

My entire family slept in one small room in a house owned by an old Mandingo man with a long, thick gray beard, whom we called old man Beard-Beard. Some believed that Beard-Beard was actually from Sinoe but had settled in Côte d'Ivoire before the war. He sold goods between Maryland County and Côte d'Ivoire. Beard-Beard was rather short and slim, and he walked erect with his head high. He was a proud, distinguished man. Our family had met Beard-Beard when we were trading palm oil across the Cavalla River between Pleebo in Maryland County and the Côte d'Ivoire side. He was one of our customers, or "custo-man," as we say in colloquial. He bought our palm oil, which we sold to him in the large five-gallon containers. It was more profitable and quicker to sell than the one-gallon containers. He bought most of our inventory on several weekly trips. I also sold gold to the old man regularly, months before we left Liberia. To reach our customers while in Côte d'Ivoire, we went to Gozon "market day" every Friday, transporting our goods in wheelbarrows.

When we arrived at the refugee camp and saw how horrible the conditions were, we went to see Beard-Beard in desperation, asking for help. He said he did not have a house to give us, so he offered us his storage room, where he stored yams. Beard-Beard had a very productive yam farm. He offered to take out the yams, store them in another location, and put *lappas* on the floor for us to sleep. *Lappas* are pieces of cotton cloth, two yards each, that women tie as skirts or around their heads. In some cultures, men also tie *lappas*. The storage room was not the most comfortable option; however, it was the only option, so we took it. We removed the yams to Beard-Beard's other warehouse, and then spent a considerable amount of time cleaning the room for our family. When we finished cleaning, the old man gave us several *lappas* for my father, mother, grandmother, and sisters. We were particularly concerned about our parents and the smaller children sleeping on *lappas* on the cold, bare floor and having to go to the toilet in the bush. We did not want them to get sick or be bitten by bugs. The rest of us—mainly my brothers and I—slept outside on Beard-Beard's market tables, barely covered with thin *lappas*. In the morning we would get up and clear the tables to help the old man prepare his market by placing his goods on the tables in a certain order. The enterprising Beard-Beard sold many products on these market tables, ranging from produce to household goods.

Gozon was a rural village like Panama. Beard-Beard's home, which he shared with his wife and daughter, was located in the middle of the village. It was a small three-bedroom house made of mud and sticks with a thatched roof. There were no windows, only open spaces or holes between mud bricks to provide ventilation. We would put pieces of cardboard boxes and *lappas* across these holes whenever it rained to prevent the floor from getting wet. We picked up odd jobs to support our family and because we wanted to get our own place quickly.

The family spent many weeks sleeping in Beard-Beard's storeroom and on top of his market tables. It seemed like an eternity, with no privacy. Going to the toilet in the bush, finding a space to defecate, digging a hole to bury feces—especially at night—was disconcerting. There could have been snakes and other pests around to bite us. We bathed in the bush as well. It was at times like these that we missed our humble home in Panama. There we had a zinc bathroom where we could wash and have some semblance of privacy. Our home also had individual rooms with beds and mattresses, as well as many windows, so we got enough ventilation.

Months after moving to Gozon, we saw that the town was overcrowding, with more and more refugees. We heard that there was another refugee camp in Tabou, a town in Côte d'Ivoire that was about ten to fifteen kilometers away, where the UNHCR agency was distributing food and other rations to refugees. Then, UNHCR started bringing food and rations to Gozon too. They gave us food, designated land for farming, and provided us with agricultural tools, such as cutlasses, hoes, diggers, and knives. They also gave us tarpaulin to cover areas for shelter or storage. We were given pots and pans, cooking utensils, and other household items. With the new tools we received, we started mining gold and farming again.

Beard-Beard offered us a corner of his yam farm where we could construct a modest house for our family. We were able to build a small house for our parents. Similar in design to our house in Panama, it was made of mud, with four bedrooms, an outside bathroom made of zinc with a *lappas* cloth door, and a kitchen that was separate from the house, located in the back. The structure was on flat land, unlike our house in Panama, which was elevated on a hill. I spearheaded the building process with my brothers' assistance. We also put up a small church, attached to the house, so our father could preach again. Although smaller than our house in Panama, with two fewer bedrooms, our new residence was large enough to accommodate our entire family. My parents, brothers, younger sisters, and I moved in. My elder sister, Agnes, and her boyfriend, Alex, built their own house nearby and accommodated some of our siblings. We now had the privacy we longed for. My brothers and I constructed the beds, including a bigger one for our parents.

In addition to helping Beard-Beard with his market and working on his yam farm, we resumed trading palm oil. In Gozon we were allowed to farm in open fields near the camp created by palm oil companies. After the companies removed the palm trees, they allowed locals to plant rice and cassava (a root plant) used to make starch, gari (farina), and fufu (a dumpling-like food that is served with hot pepper soup and an assortment of meat, chicken, and fish). We were not allowed to plant any other crops. Having previously owned a farm in Liberia, the Nyenswah clan took advantage of the opportunity to plant rice and cassava. Our farm became quite productive. We fed our family and sold the surplus produce in the market. My brothers and I dug gold in the nearby mine, though farming was a better and easier option. The Decoris Oil Palm Company in Pleebo, from which we bought oil in Pleebo, was abandoned when rebel leaders illegally seized their palm farms. Palm oil was in demand, so we traded ours with the rebels for other food items and household goods or sold it to them when the price was good.

These people we called rebels were mostly young teenage boys, with a few girls at times, who had been recruited by force by rebel group leaders—either by threatening their lives or actually killing their parents or other family members right before their very eyes to prove that resistance could be fatal. Often, these boys were drugged with one substance or another and made to kill people as a show of strength and willingness to follow the leader. They were trained to be ruthless in every respect. They did not take no for an answer. Some of them were as young as we were, some even younger. Several had been snatched from their families or caught in the bush while attempting to escape the onslaught of rebel gangs in their villages and towns. It was easy doing business with them because we had prior experience trading with rebels in Liberia. We knew their needs and wants: clothing, food, and small radios to play the music of Lucky Dube, a South African reggae musician and Rastafarian. These guys loved Lucky Dube. His music was used as their anthem or call to arms, depending on the chosen song of the day.

Gozon refugee camp was as far as we could travel, as Côte d'Ivoire did not allow refugees to settle in their urban cities. The war and the long strenuous expedition south had interrupted my education. I had been out of school for three years, displaced with my family. Regardless, my education remained a primary family goal. As a Methodist minister, my father had contacts that extended across national boundaries. He knew Rev. Humphrey C. Kumeh, who lived in Tabou with his family. Reverend Kumeh was a Methodist pastor from Greenville, where he had worked for an American Methodist missionary, Nancy Lightfoot, translating the New Testament Bible from English into Kru. The Kumehs were prominent in Greenville and considered wealthy by most people. They too had been forced to migrate to Côte d'Ivoire as refugees, though they had settled earlier on and were now living a rather good, productive life. My father made arrangements for me to board with Reverend Kumeh and his wife, Munah, in their home in Tabou. By moving to Tabou, I could go to school at no cost because the refugee schools did not charge tuition. Students only needed a place to live.

So, in 1995, two years after we settled in Gozon, my father took me to Tabou. I was heartbroken to leave my parents, brothers, and sisters again for yet another unfamiliar experience. I was uncertain what the conditions would be in my new situation. I definitely did not want to undergo similar hardships as I had experienced with the Russ family. But we all had to adapt. My parents would stay in Gozon until July 1999. It was the place our family called home and the foreign land where we made new friends.

The Kumehs' home was a mid-sized three-bedroom house with a living room, dining room, bathroom, and indoor kitchen. I slept on the floor in the living room. Residing with the Kumehs felt like living with the Russ family, much to my chagrin. I had similar chores. I had to wash and press clothes for the entire family, cut wood, make a fire for cooking and heating water, clean the house and yard, and go to the market. I did all this, and other assigned chores, in exchange for my board, even though I had no room of my own.

Rice was the staple food, but on many occasions we ate bulgur wheat instead because so many of us refugee children lived with the Kumehs. Feeding all of us must have been quite an undertaking. Although I knew I was poor, I felt even poorer in this environment. I had no clothes, no shoes, and no money. I would see my peers playing football and having fun, and I wished I could have joined them. Yet, I could not. They did not want me around because I was penniless. They laughed at me and called me horrible names, like "jackass" or "slave." They said I was not good enough to play with them because I was "working for people as a houseboy." Some said I was raggedy because my clothes were old and tattered, although they were clean, and I did not have body odor as some people did. Hence, I kept to myself to avoid being belittled. I went to school, studied hard to ace all my subjects, learned as much as I could, and prayed for the day when I would not be called poor again.

Remarkably, my high school days in Tabou were some of my best. We had exceptional teachers compared to the instructors at a typical high school in Liberia. Most of them were professionals with master's or doctoral degrees, who themselves were refugees. They often could not get jobs in their professional areas while displaced, so most of them resorted to teaching high school. There was only one English-language high school in Tabou. All others were French-language institutions, as Côte d'Ivoire is a Francophone country that had been colonized by the French. We had expatriate teachers, too, from various English-speaking countries. Most of the Liberian refugees went to the English-language school.

At school, there was a meal program. They gave us cooked meals consisting of beans, rice, soup, wheat, and other foods, thanks to UNHCR and ADRA, which had established and ran the school. This food kept us going throughout the day. I particularly welcomed the program. It meant I had a full stomach and would not have to worry about whether I had enough to eat when I got home, where there were so many people sharing a limited amount of food.

In school I met Gyude Moore and Snoh Myers, two boys from Liberia, and we became good friends. Gyude was from Maryland County and Snoh was from Sinoe like me, though we never met in Sinoe. Snoh and I also shared a desk in our very cramped refugee classroom. The three of us studied English together. Snoh was just as poor as I was. Gyude was not poor, and unlike the others, he actually treated me warmly in spite of my situation. I was grateful to have him as a companion. Being around him made me see the light at the end of the tunnel. I began to believe in myself once more and prayed even harder that the day would soon come when my life would change for the better—as my parents envisioned and always reminded me. Poverty would be a thing in my past.

The refugee high school was a fifteen-minute walk from the Kumehs' house. It had excellent administrators and was well managed. The school was a three-story concrete building, enclosed in a fence to protect and restrict students from leaving school grounds. The classrooms were spacious and could easily accommodate at least thirty to forty students each. Every classroom had mounted blackboards and wooden desks, which were locally made. Because of the large number of students, annexes were constructed adjacent to the school building. They were makeshift structures with thatched roofs and walls. My eleventh-grade class took place in an annex.

I was very active in high school. Though I was mocked for being poor, my classmates respected me because I was smart. My major subjects were science and mathematics. I excelled in the sciences—chemistry, biology, physics, and mathematics. I also excelled in English. My grades were usually in the 90%–100% range, though I struggled to get through French and social studies.

I was a member of the student council government and liaised with the school administration and faculty on behalf of students. I also spoke to UNHCR and ADRA, championing the rights of refugee students. My involvement in student affairs gave me the opportunity to develop strong, long-lasting friendships. I was speaker of my class in both years, as well as a member of the Press Club, which required me to write many articles about a range of issues affecting refugees in Côte d'Ivoire. I wrote about the lives of refugees, student behavior, rights of children, and the UN system—in particular, UNHCR. I was interviewed by a BBC News team to discuss the plight of refugee students in Côte d'Ivoire. I advocated for the rights of refugees, speaking numerous times on the school radio, which was known as the Voice of Tabou 11 (VOTT). I wanted to raise awareness about these issues to better the lives of refugees in Tabou.

I was arrested for my outspokenness. Police officers would frequently harass refugees, demanding that we show our papers and identity cards. Sometimes on weekends I traveled from Tabou to Gozon to visit my family. There were several checkpoints guarded by Ivorian police and immigration officers. The first thing they asked for was my immigration papers. Refugees were never given papers. It was always embarrassing. During one of my travels, the immigration officer recognized me. I was arrested and interrogated but later released through the intervention of Reverend Kumeh.

One hot day in October 1994 I went to the soccer field near the Kumehs' house. Due to the Kumehs' strict rules, I would not venture out often. Going to the field was my only solace because there I could play with other children and have a good time. I loved soccer. It was my favorite pastime next to reading. Like any other day, boys from the refugee neighborhood were out for soccer practice. On the other end of the field, there was a group of young girls playing kickball. I spotted this girl, distinct from the crowd. She was so beautiful. She moved with such grace on the field, running to kick and score a goal. When she scored, she jumped for joy. Her goal broke the tie in the game. Her team won. Bravo! I knew that I wanted to get close to this girl, who was not only lovely but could also play kickball well! I wondered how I could meet her.

I discovered she lived near the soccer field, close to the Kumehs' home. Thereafter, I watched for her every morning and waited to see her as she walked to school in her pretty outfits. I noticed that she went to the soccer field for kickball practice on most days after school. I was so intrigued by her. It appeared that she was devoted to school, completing her daily studies before going to play in the field.

I learned her name through my friend Harrison Togba, Reverend Kumeh's nephew who also lived with the Kumehs. Harrison was a few years older than I and much more experienced. When I told Harrison that I could not stop thinking about this girl, he laughed because he knew her and her family quite well. Her name was Josephine. She was also a refugee. She was born in Harper City, Maryland County. Her father had migrated from Grand Kru County and settled in Harper City, where he later married her mother, Beatrice, and raised his family. It was common in those days for the Krus to travel from their rural communities to Harper City in search of a better education and exposure to a wider society, so many people put down roots there.

Geographically, Grand Kru shares a border with Maryland County on the east, River Gee County in the north, and Sinoe in the west. Grebo, the language spoken in Maryland and River Gee Counties, is very similar to Kru, which made it easier for Kru people to migrate to these places. The Kru language is also spoken in parts of Maryland County, so in essence, Josephine and I would speak the same language.

Harrison offered to introduce me. He said that he would go to Josephine's house and tell her about me beforehand. Several weeks later Harrison and I walked toward Josephine on the soccer field. We took a seat behind a Sekou Toure medicine tree, from which many herbs were collected and used for treatment by traditional medicine men. When Josephine saw us, she smiled and looked at me as if to ask, "Is this your friend?" Harrison greeted her and introduced me.

In a shy voice, Josephine said, "Pleased to meet you, Tolbert."

"I'm also glad to meet you, Josephine," I answered.

We exchanged pleasantries and then she left, avoiding eye contact with me as she walked away.

I felt inferior and belittled. I did not live with my own parents. I lived in a home where I was considered domestic help. My father had limited education and my mother never went to school. We were poor. I was not in Josephine's social class. Nevertheless, I knew I would one day rise above a life of poverty and deprivation and be the man my father said I would become.

Harrison started visiting Josephine to talk about me and tell her how much I loved her. She told him she was neither interested in a friendship nor a romantic relationship because I was too poor. She said that I looked like a suffering and neglected child. I wasn't presentable. I had no money and was too destitute to buy her fancy things as the other boys did for their girlfriends. She rejected me for months, despite Harrison's constant interventions. The more he persisted, the more she remained firm. She said I was too poor, I did not live with my own parents, I was a refugee house servant. And she was right. I had nothing except my love and devotion to give her.

Harrison knew that Josephine was having difficulties with her science classes and that I happened to be exceptionally talented in those subjects. He suggested that I help her with science and math classes, so I began visiting her home after school to tutor her. As time passed, Josephine discovered that I was a good teacher and her grades began improving. She discovered I was a good-hearted person with a determination to succeed in life. She noticed that I stayed focused on my schooling despite my suffering and observed that I was a strong debater. Slowly Josephine developed a liking for me. Yet the more I stated my feelings for her, the more she rejected me. One day, months after our tutoring sessions began, the tide turned and Josephine decided to give me a try. She, an eighth grader, said she saw "potential" in me. We started courting secretly, hiding from her parents and the Kumehs. Only Harrison knew.

Josephine lived with both of her parents and her six siblings. Before the war, they had lived in Harper City, where their home was a well-constructed, two-story concrete building. In Tabou, her father, Mr. Kikeh, had rented a one-bedroom unit with a porch in a concrete building that had six other one-bedroom apartments. There were no individual bathrooms or kitchens. Mr. Kikeh had built a partially open tent that was used as the family kitchen and constructed a bathroom made of palm branches and sticks outside of the house, which he covered with a cloth door. Josephine and her sisters slept in the room that operated as the living room during the day.

Mr. Kikeh kept a watchful eye over his children, particularly the girls. I was only able to see Josephine at her home when I tutored her and even then, only when Mr. Kikeh was away. Mrs. Kikeh was a businesswoman who traveled between Côte d'Ivoire and Grand Kru and the gold-mining camp to sell an assortment of goods, including used clothes and food. She had been in business before the war and was the family's primary breadwinner after they migrated to Ivory Coast. As a result, she was absent much of the time. Mr. Kikeh had been a well-known electrician in Harper City. Despite steady employment, Mr. Kikeh could not provide for his growing family on his salary alone so he joined his wife selling peanuts, bananas, candles, and other products on small market tables. The Kikehs were not considered rich, yet they were not considered poor either, as they maintained a semblance of economic stability. Mrs. Kikeh was considered quite successful. Consequently, Josephine's living standards were much higher than mine, and her family was considered middle class by refugee standards.

Josephine had more freedom than other teenagers. She was well dressed and wore fancy clothes, with nice shoes and handbags to match. She had money to go out with her friends. Harrison said that Josephine was embarrassed to be seen with me because my clothes were threadbare, and I did not have the means to take her out to the places she wanted to go. She felt she could not justify to her friends why she would want to go out with me, especially when all of their boyfriends were taking them to fine establishments. They took their girlfriends to the movies, gave them money, and bought them lovely things. No matter how hard Harrison and I tried, Josephine refused to be seen with me publicly, except when we walked to school in the morning or met on the soccer field in the evening.

One thing that deepened my love for Josephine was her reserved nature. She did not run around with as many boys as her friends did. Boys who bragged about what they did or didn't do with girls had nothing negative to say about Josephine. They only said that she played hard to get. I myself had experienced this! It took months for her to even agree to be my friend—she was that particular. But I knew she was a respectful girl and one day I would take her home to meet my mother.

Harrison, who earned a satisfactory living as the manager of the poultry store owned by the Methodist church, came up with a plan that would allow me to spend time alone with Josephine. He invited her to go to a local restaurant for *achekeh*, a popular Ivorian dish. *Achekeh* is made from fermented cassava, which is then ground and pounded, refined into a grain similar to couscous or farina. The tasty dish is usually served with onion gravy, and sometimes with roasted fish or chicken, fried plantain, cucumber salad, and hot pepper on the side. We all loved *achekeh*!

The three of us met under the Sekou Toure medicine tree and walked to the restaurant and picked up three fish-and-*achekeh* meals. After buying the food, Harrison told us we would take it to a place where we could all sit and talk. He had rented a room in a motel not far from where we lived. I was a naive country boy who never would have dared to be so bold. It was out of the ordinary for me, but Harrison felt that we needed a moment of privacy together.

When we arrived at the motel, Josephine was surprised.

"Why are we in a motel?" she asked.

"Because we can all sit and talk in a more relaxed atmosphere, as we can't take you to our house. My uncle and aunt would have a fit!" Harrison said.

I saw her embarrassment. Like me, this was also the first time Josephine had ever entered a motel. The room was very small. However, I was grateful that it had its own bathroom. Thank God it was not outside! No one could see us going to the bathroom! I also noticed that the room had no windows.

Right after we finished eating, Harrison excused himself, saying that he had to check on something at work. I could not believe I was finally alone in a private room with the girl I loved. It was awkward at first—very awkward, indeed. We tried to make small talk. She was shy and uneasy, and I was too. I told her that I would not take advantage of her just because we were alone. We continued talking, then I gently pulled her toward me and kissed her: first on the cheek, then on the lips. To my astonishment, she responded with pleasure. She, too, wanted to be kissed. In the heat of the moment, we shared an intimate experience for the first time.

The next week Josephine refused to see me. She avoided going to our usual meeting places. She left home earlier to avoid walking to school with me. She told Harrison that she was ashamed. I wanted to see her to let her know that I was not going anywhere. I knew she was the girl for me: the one I would marry. After this talk, she felt more comfortable about our relationship and began visiting me at the Kumehs' house after school. One day Mrs. Kumeh came in earlier than expected and saw Josephine in the house and asked her point-blank what she was doing there. "I came to see Tolbert," she whispered. Mrs. Kumeh responded, "Don't come back here again, or I will tell your father." The possibility of her father knowing about our relationship frightened Josephine; yet she could not stay away from me nor could I stay away from her. We confided in Harrison and he came up with another clever plan.

This time he planned to visit Josephine, knowing that her father knew him through Mr. Kumeh, who was Harrison's uncle and Mr. Kikeh's friend. Harrison became more familiar with her family through these frequent visits. One day Mr. Kikeh said to him, "I am not pleased that you visit my daughter all the time. What are your intentions?" Harrison then confessed: "It is my friend Tolbert Nyenswah who likes Josephine, and I am only talking to Josephine to get her interested in Tolbert. This boy really loves your daughter, Mr. Kikeh. He is very serious about her, and he is a good person."

"Then he must come to the house himself if he likes her that much. I want to see who this Tolbert Nyenswah is. In fact, he must come with his parents so we can know his family," demanded Mr. Kikeh.

"What parents?" I asked Harrison. "My parents don't even live in Tabou. I can't ask Reverend Kumeh and his wife to come and meet Mr. Kikeh and pretend he's my father when I am sleeping on his living room floor and serving his family. He will think I am crazy. A poor boy like me wants to court a girl like Josephine? It won't work."

Without better options, Harrison canceled the proposed meeting.

Gradually, Mr. Kikeh became less strict, and I was invited to visit his home with Harrison. Getting to know Mr. Kikeh was difficult. I was afraid of the man, but Harrison kept me focused on winning Josephine. Mr. Kikeh insisted that if I wanted to visit his daughter, I had to bring my parents to meet her family. Harrison suggested that we tell Mr. Kikeh the truth and not waste his time. So, I told Mr. Kikeh my parents were Liberian refugees living in Gozon, that my father was a Methodist pastor, and that we lived a stable life until the war displaced us. I told him that I came to live with the Kumehs because I wanted to go to high school.

"Then you have to bring Reverend Kumeh to meet my family," he said.

Harrison and I did not take Reverend Kumeh to meet Mr. Kikeh. I never once considered mentioning this situation to the Kumehs. But, as time went by, the Kikeh family became acquainted with me, and I was welcomed into their home and allowed to visit at reasonable hours.

One of Josephine's chores was to cook the main family meal every day. She started saving food for me whenever she cooked, and I would come to her house after school to eat with her. This made me happy because it meant I had at least one decent meal to eat every day. During this time, Mr. Kikeh became friendlier. But Josephine's sister, Annie, did not like me at all. She saw me in my worn clothing and thought that I was not good enough for her sister and that I should not be allowed to be seen with her, especially in public. Annie told Josephine that I was too poor to do anything for her and so she had no business liking me. Being the eldest daughter and eight years older than Josephine, she even became angry with her father for agreeing to meet with me and for accepting me into his home. She insisted that I couldn't do anything for myself and if I got Josephine pregnant, it would be bad news for the entire family. The other siblings held similar views but they were not as vocal as Annie. As Josephine's big sister, with a lot more experience with boys, I believe, Annie was only being protective of her little sister and wanted only the best for her.

When Mrs. Kikeh returned to Tabou from a business trip, she got an earful from Annie and the other children. Without meeting me, she formed a negative opinion of me. She did not want a poor boy anywhere near Josephine, and she did not hide her feelings.

Beatrice Kikeh was a fair-skinned woman, who stood about five feet, six inches tall. She had large sleepy eyes, a slender face, and full lips. Her hair was jet black—long, thick, and shining. Her skin had a healthy glow that made her look golden. Beatrice was a charismatic and affectionate mother, a smooth-talking and easygoing woman, yet always firm in her decisions. She had never learned to read, though she possessed street smarts and an excellent mind for business. As a child, when she realized that her family in Grand Kru was too poor to pay for her school fees, she spent her time preparing a market and sold raw and roasted peanuts, bananas, oranges, peanut candy, coconut candy, fried plantains, and an assortment of other small items to generate income to help herself and her family. She supported her entire family this way and sent her younger brothers and sisters to school. She forfeited her own education so that they would have a better chance of living a life free of destitution. Beatrice's business had continued to expand throughout her adulthood and marriage.

Between Annie and her mother, Josephine was pressured every day to stop seeing me. However, no matter what they did or said or how badly they made her feel, Josephine cared for me and refused to let me go.

Harrison and I decided to move into our own room in a boardinghouse. Since it was a single room, we worked out an arrangement to accommodate each other in this cramped space. Whenever one person had a visitor, the other person would make himself scarce and sleep at a friend's nearby home. We had our mattress on the cement floor. The bathroom was outside. We split the monthly rent. I got a part-time job with MSF, digging latrines and wells for the refugee communities. This was very hard labor, and Josephine certainly did not want her boyfriend to be a toilet-digger, so I became an after-school tutor. I taught children every day in five or six different homes. I was also a tutor for Patricia, Josephine's youngest sister. My earnings went from 5,000 CFA to 20,000 CFA per month (US$100), which was enough to pay my rent and buy food.

Six months after Mr. Kikeh invited me into his home and blessed my friendship with his daughter, I took Josephine to meet my parents and siblings. It was a Friday evening when we left Tabou on a forty-five-minute bus ride to Gozon. The roads were dusty and dangerous, and there were two dozen people seated in the minibus, with others standing in the aisle. On many occasions minibuses have been involved in accidents on the Tabou-Gozon highway, which is a terrible route with dilapidated bridges. Harrison and I experienced this one weekend when we were traveling to see my parents in Gozon. We never arrived in Gozon and had to return to Tabou on another bus that met us at the site of the accident.

My mother was waiting when we stepped off the bus, and she greeted Josephine warmly. We went to my parents' house to meet my father and the rest of the family. My brothers were at the gold mines. My sisters and their children and others all stopped by to meet Josephine. Everyone was happy to see us. After spending an hour or so with my parents, we went to greet my cousins who lived in the house next door. It was thrilling to see my family after being away from them for two long years. Because this was the first time that I had brought over a girlfriend, they treated Josephine remarkably well. Here I was, all the way from Tabou, not alone but with a girl I loved whom I wanted them to meet. They knew she had to be special, and Josephine felt that way immediately because my family embraced her at the onset. There was no opposition to her or my relationship with her. Everyone accepted her, and in an instant, she knew that she had her own special relationship with me. My brothers arrived home from the mines just in time to meet Josephine before we left for the bus depot. It was pure joy seeing them again, even more so because they embraced Josephine as warmly as my mother had.

But Annie continued to press her mother, making it clear that I should never become a part of their family. Mrs. Kikeh agreed. Again, they ordered Josephine to leave me. She refused. When her friends joined the chorus of displeasure, her mother and Annie tried to discourage her even more. This was the complete opposite of my family's reception of Josephine, and they had met her only once. What was apparent, however, was that her friends—who had all the things that money could buy—were jealous of Josephine's poor but caring and committed boyfriend. They began to stay away from her and refused to spend time with her, which only made Josephine more determined to be with me. She told her friends, "I see him for myself, and I make my own decisions. Tolbert loves and cares for me. He does whatever he can for me, and I am grateful to have him in my life."

Her resolve caused a rift in the family, which upset her greatly. Despite the household tension, nothing could sway her. With the pressure mounting, I told her that she should leave me because I could not yet provide for her and did not want her to abandon her loved ones. Josephine responded, "I will not leave you. I believe in you and I love you. I am prepared to take my chance with you." She started clinging to me and acted as if she owned me. She made me do everything with her. This possessive shift bothered me, but I knew that she became insecure due to the situation with her family. I was patient because I knew undoubtedly that she was devoted to me and that is what I wanted—a girl who would be as devoted to me as I was to her.

As Josephine bickered with her sister and mother, I developed trust with her father. He knew that my intentions were honorable and that I truly cared for her, so when the Kikehs moved back to their home in Harper City with their other children in 1996, he asked me to look after Josephine. They left Josephine so she could finish tenth grade in Tabou before joining them in Liberia. When the family left, I moved into the house with her. I felt that the freedom for which I had long waited was coming gradually. We lived together like a married couple. We cooked, ate, and slept together in the same room every night. But I knew that staying with Josephine was inappropriate since we were not married, and cohabitation was against our Christian upbringing.

In 1997, at the age of twenty-three, I graduated from high school. After spending many of my teenage years roaming from place to place and missing out on academia, I felt truly accomplished. The event was singularly festive. Ivorian government officials attended the ceremony. We gave speeches, sang songs, and marched down the streets of Tabou.

That same year, Charles Taylor won the first postwar election, becoming president of Liberia. After the election, Liberia appeared to have achieved peace. The war seemed to be over. Everything the Nyenswahs heard from family and friends who had remained in Liberia indicated that serenity was at hand.

UNHCR announced that only refugees who wanted to return to Liberia would be repatriated. I desperately wanted to go to college, but it was feasible in Côte d'Ivoire only for those who spoke French fluently. There was no English-speaking university. Although I had passed the college entrance exam for refugee students, the only way I could further my education was to return to Liberia. And so I signed up with UNHCR for voluntary repatriation. This meant leaving Josephine, with the promise that I would send for her when my situation improved. Saying goodbye to my family, yet again, was difficult.

I left Côte d'Ivoire in 1997 on a UNHCR truck loaded with refugees. We spent two days on rugged roads to get to Monrovia via Nimba County. Meanwhile, Josephine returned to Harper City to live with her parents and finish high school.

Why am I so passionate about this woman? I asked myself. *Am I sure that I want her to be my wife?* The more questions I considered, the more convinced I was that Josephine was the girl for me.

And why is that? I wondered again.

The answers came easily: Josephine is wonderful. There is no doubt about that. She is unique. No doubt about that. She is worldly. She is devoted to me. She is caring and encouraging. She will support me in my quest for upward mobility. She is no longer uncomfortable with my humble village background. She is an African woman with a clear understanding of an African woman's stature and conduct. She will care for me, build a home with me, and together we will have and raise beautiful children.

I assured Josephine that as soon as I settled in Monrovia with a job and a room of my own, I would send for her. Comforted by my promise, she said she would wait for me.

CHAPTER 5

Total Collapse of Public Health Care Services

The Ebola virus disease (EVD) outbreak led to significant declines in utilization of health services from August to December 2014, compared to the same period in 2012 and 2013.[1] These declines were partly due to temporary closures of health facilities and partly because of lower attendance due to mistrust of the health system. Those who made it to health facilities were often shunned and were not attended, even women in labor, because of the fear of Ebola; some even died as a result. With limited access to public sector health facilities, where services were normally provided free, out-of-pocket spending increased due to use of alternative services, further limiting access to services. Morbidity rates increased, and mortality rates reversed any gains that had been made.

In early August, the CDC team lead, Dr. Kevin De Cock, proposed to me that we consider establishing an incident management system (IMS), based on the CDC model for emergency response. The IMS, I was told, "is a standardized tool for responding to emergencies, under which personnel and resources are organized and managed around specific objectives. It focuses financial and logistics in support of specific scientific and public health objectives."[2] I wondered why Dr. De Cock proposed this to me instead of to Minister of Health Walter Gwenigale or my immediate boss, Bernice Dahn, the chief medical officer (CMO). They were in charge of the national coordination.

The Médecins Sans Frontières (MSF) team had expressed its dismay at the indecision and inaction on the part of the government. They wanted the minister and CMO to be more decisive and act more quickly on the specifics of the response. Under the leadership of Dr. De Cock, the CDC team made an early recommendation to the Ministry of Health to restrict the number of attendees at the Ebola task force meetings, but on any given day there were close to one hundred people in the room. People who did not need to be there, or had no business being there, were often present. The meetings became a free-for-all, open to the public. There was neither follow-up to ensure that proposed actions were implemented nor any reporting system in place to track implementation, the degree of implementation, and whether or not the implemented action could be considered successful. Meetings tended to start late and ran overtime.

Representatives of both MSF and the CDC saw enthusiasm in what I was doing as head of Social Mobilization, engaging the community, interacting with the local and foreign media, and handling dead body management. I was seen everywhere in Monrovia and heard on the radio everywhere in Liberia. Liberians were saying, "Tolbert Nyenswah is all over the place."

The national coordination team was recommended by WHO representative Dr. Nestor Ndayimirije, who was very apprehensive about the CDC's recommendation of a new coordination structure, instead of the task force that was already in place. But the National Task Force had deferred its oversight responsibilities to others—specifically, international partner organizations that came to help in the response, who seemed to be running the show. This had prompted the national legislature and the Liberian public to voice their lack of confidence in the Ministry of Health's ability to handle the response.

At a meeting chaired by Minister Gwenigale, with CMO Dahn and other officials of government in attendance, the CDC staff proposed to the ministry that an incident management system be established, with one incident manager who would be given overall responsibility for Liberia's national Ebola response. I was present in that meeting, taking notes attentively. CMO Dahn was convinced that this would clearly define roles and authority and foster accountability, making management of the response more efficient. The IMS would become the technical coordinating body for the multinational, intersectoral partners and assistance that was now starting to come into the country. As the technical coordinating body, the IMS would determine how response strategies were implemented, at national, county, and emergency operation centers across Liberia.

The CDC recommended that the task force focus on restoring the health care delivery system, which was collapsing. It seemed that practically all health care delivery facilities stopped functioning when Ebola struck.

The health system was ill equipped to effectively respond to the epidemic with the necessary occupational health and safety and infection prevention and control (IPC) measures for safe and effective health services. As a result, health workers were suffering a 30 times higher risk of infection compared to the general population. By April 8, 2015, a total of 372 health workers were infected, of whom 184 died.[1] Preexisting structural vulnerabilities included inadequately trained health workers who were also insufficient in numbers and poorly motivated; infrastructure and equipment were unsuitable, supply chains were weak, and the quality of care was poor. This led to disruptions in the delivery of routine health services with health facility closures, fears and refusal of health workers to provide routine health services, and community mistrust and fear. Coverage of life-saving maternal and child health interventions, in particular, declined dramatically. Even in the midst of the outbreak, there was a need to rebuild the health system.

Pregnant women had no place to deliver their babies. Immunization services closed down, and people were dying in the streets. The United Nations Population Fund (UNFPA) published a story titled "Pregnant in the Shadow of Ebola: Deteriorating Health Systems Endanger

Women," underscoring the experience of Comfort Fayiah, a thirty-six-year-woman who encountered major obstacles searching for a medical facility to deliver her baby during the height of the Ebola crisis. In the words of her husband, Victor Fayiah, "we went to four different clinics and hospitals, but they would not allow my wife in. I begged them, I cried, but they bluntly refused." Instead of receiving care from hospital staff, "she was assisted by people on the streets, some of whom shielded her from the nearby traffic." Victor Fayiah went on to say that "onlookers came, including women who formed a human chain barrier using their clothes, while a nurse assistant, who was passing on a motorbike, assisted my wife to deliver." Ultimately, Comfort Fayiah delivered twin girls.[3] The plight of this woman in this story could be reverberated by numerous other women throughout the country. I found myself in the thick of things when my phone started ringing twenty-four seven, particularly at night, with calls from women in desperate search of urgent care. They voiced complaints of being refused care due to a lack of hospital beds, being charged exorbitant fees in public hospitals that were supposed to provide care free of charge, or ambulance services to take them to the hospital was not available.

Prior to the Ebola epidemic, health workers had initiated two strike actions. They had voiced their discontent with the leadership of the health sector in Liberia and had several misunderstandings with the Ministry of Health authorities. The discontent related mainly to poor conditions of work; not being paid well, with long lapses between payments; inadequate equipment and supplies in hospitals; facilities that were in disrepair; and a lack of confidence in the administration of the Ministry of Health. Now, they were refusing to work because, in addition to not being paid well or on time, they had no personal protective equipment, there were no IPC measures in place to care for Ebola patients, and there was a lack of running water and electricity in major health facilities.

On August 8, President Ellen Johnson Sirleaf convened a meeting at the Monrovia City Hall with close to three hundred health care workers from all health facilities in Monrovia to discuss their concerns. The meeting occurred in the theater of the City Hall, which had a maximum seating capacity of three hundred ninety-eight, according to City Hall officials. The theater was overcrowded. Health workers stood shoulder to shoulder against other officials of government. I was sitting at the back, taking notes. The president's intention, amidst the crisis, was to re-open health facilities that had been abandoned. The meeting was intense. Hostile remarks were made against the ministry's leadership by representatives of the health workforce. It was an unfriendly atmosphere, and the meeting ended without resolution of the problems.

The next day, President Sirleaf visited Minister Gwenigale for further discussions on resolving the health workforce crisis. According to Minister Gwenigale, the president requested that someone other than the minister and CMO be designated to manage the Ebola response team, and that restoration of health services should be separated from response activities. The minister stated that the president mentioned me, by name, as the person she had in mind to manage the response. Minister Gwenigale said he was astonished!

Nevertheless, at the president's behest, Minister Gwenigale requested a meeting with me the next morning, August 10. At that meeting, with apparent reluctance, Gwenigale told me, "I don't know why the president says I should separate the response from restoration of health services. She came here yesterday and named you as the one who should be in charge of the Ebola response." The minister looked perplexed.

I was shocked. I had never even had a one-on-one conversation with the president.

Minister Gwenigale continued, "The president said I should remove Chief Medical Officer Dahn, who has been leading the response, and have her restore health care services by getting the health workers back to work. But I want to talk to you and Dr. Dahn tomorrow."

The following day, Dr. Dahn and I met with the minister, who repeated what he had told me. Interestingly, though not surprising, Dr. Dahn said, "I trust this man. He is competent to lead the response."

I was silent for a moment, taking time for all this to sink in. Then I asked the minister to officially write to me, clearly stating what the president had instructed him to do. On August 11, I was officially put in charge of Liberia's Ebola response as incident manager and chair of the IMS. As such, I remained in my position as assistant minister for preventive services. However, my responsibilities were delegated to my colleague, Dr. Saye Baawo (now deceased), who was assistant minister for curative services. I asked Minister Gwenigale to introduce me to the many partners and international responders at the meeting that he or the CMO chaired every morning.

The appointment was not without risks. It could either make or break me and alter the course of my career. I was an assistant minister, a junior in the government's ministerial hierarchy. Now, suddenly, I would be directing the activities of many more-senior government officials, not only from Liberia but the United Nations and other international agencies. This was a huge responsibility. There were many within the ministry who were most displeased that I had been chosen. Some were unapologetically angry. Yet I knew that I had the capacity to do the job. And I recognized that the honor of being selected to such a unique leadership role in our nation's history was a dream my father had the day I was born. He had said this was my destiny, and he had believed wholeheartedly that his prediction would come to pass while I was relatively young. He said that, when the time came, I would recognize the calling and be prepared to take the charge. Remembering the words of my father, with humility and resolve, I accepted the responsibility bestowed upon me by the president to serve as incident manager and chairman of the IMS, to fight the Ebola outbreak in Liberia.

Leading the IMS was unprecedented for someone who had started working at the MOHSW as a secretary. When I arrived in Monrovia from Côte d'Ivoire, the city was in a dismal state. It was 1997, the year Charles Taylor won the presidential election. After several years of chaotic, stop-and-go fighting, I thought that the war was over for good. That exuberant feeling would be short-lived.

Monrovia had no electricity, no running water, no fancy buildings. Even rustic Tabou had lights and running water. I had heard that the Ivory Coast's economic capital of Abidjan was a bustling city with fine homes and elegant architecture. Daily life functioned smoothly. That was how I expected Monrovia to be. Instead, it looked like a slum. The roads were deplorable, worse than the roads in my village in Panama. People drew water from wells. The electrical grid and hydroelectric dam had been destroyed and looted during the war. Poverty was rampant. Conditions seemed worse than in Panama or Tabou—particularly astonishing when one considers that I was a very poor refugee there, with tattered clothes and no shoes. Monrovia was filthy. There was garbage everywhere, even near the government office buildings. People often remarked that many of these buildings had terrible odors due to the lack of running water to flush toilets. People would flush with water they carried in buckets. When the buckets or water storage barrels were empty, people used the toilets without flushing. The stench at the entrance to some of these government office buildings was putrid.

I lived with my uncle Robert, who had a house in New Kru Town, a northwestern coastal suburb of Monrovia. As four other boys lived there, I slept on the floor in a single room at the back of the house. I desperately wanted to go to college, but attending college required money. So, I found a job in the capitol building, the seat of the National Legislature, as the page for the Sinoe County senator, the Honorable Harrison Slewion (now deceased). "You carry the bags and do whatever needs to be done," he told me. I followed him around, carrying his briefcase, doing chores, and serving as his messenger and errand boy. The work reminded me of working for the Russes and Kumehs, but it was a means to an end and I performed my job with humility.

I found a second job teaching math and science at the Meal-A-Day School in Point Four on Bushrod Island, in New Kru Town, where I lived. I worked there for nearly a year, earning 500 Liberian dollars per month, equivalent to about US$12.50 at the time. The additional income gave me enough to buy basic necessities such as toothpaste and soap, as well as have a few Liberian dollars in my pocket. I used the money from my job with Senator Slewion to live on and put a little aside every month toward my college education.

One day in the senator's office I met Stephen T. Tweh, who worked at the MOHSW. Mr. Tweh was the special assistant to the Honorable Arthur A. D. Saye, deputy minister of health for administration and the brother-in-law of President Taylor. He was also Senator Slevion's friend from Sinoe High School. I asked Mr. Tweh if he knew of any jobs in his office. I told him I was a high school graduate and that while in Côte d'Ivoire I had studied computer science. Being computer literate in the 1990s in a country like Liberia was a big deal. Mr. Tweh smiled broadly as he told me that they had a computer in their office, but no one knew how to operate it. He invited me to take a look.

At six o'clock the following morning, I was outside Mr. Tweh's house in New Kru Town to ride with him to work. His driver pulled up in a white pickup truck; I sat in the back of the truck while he sat in the front seat with the driver, who stopped multiple times to pick up MOHSW workers along the way.

At the ministry, Mr. Tweh introduced me to Deputy Minister Saye and recommended me for a job helping the staff use computers. At the ministry, 99.9% of the employees were using typewriters, while their computers were covered up with a white cloth. Apparently, the Israeli government had donated these computers but most of the staff was computer illiterate. The offices of the minister of health, deputy minister of health for administration, deputy minister of health / chief medical officer, deputy minister of health for planning, and deputy minister of social welfare all had computers that were sitting on desks, covered up.

In Deputy Minister Saye's office, I removed the cloth and turned on the computer. I requested that they give me documents to be typed and printed from the computer. The entire day, I typed and printed so many documents for Mr. Tweh. People came around from other offices to see what I was doing. They were amazed! When the letters were printed and taken to Deputy Minister Saye, he invited me into his office, where he interviewed me and hired me on the spot as a secretary. In addition,

I was asked to conduct orientation and tutoring in basic computer literacy for other secretaries in the building. This was the beginning of my employment with the MOHSW.

New Kru Town was roughly thirteen miles from the MOHSW, which made getting to and from work a major challenge. I did not have a vehicle, and Monrovia had a very limited public transportation system at the time. Fortunately, I discovered that another employee at the ministry also lived in New Kru Town and owned a four-door cabin pickup truck with an open back. I offered to help him clean his truck every morning in exchange for a ride to work. There was no seat for me in the cabin, so I rode in the back of the pickup truck. If I was running late and missed my ride, I had to walk several miles from New Kru Town to the Gabriel Tucker Bridge, where I could catch a local bus.

In 1999 I passed the University of Liberia entrance examination. With the help of a merit scholarship from the United Methodist Church, I enrolled in the science college, majoring in biology, with a minor in chemistry. My dream was to become a medical doctor.

A year after enrolling in university, I wrote to Josephine and invited her to join me in Monrovia. It had been three long years since we were last together. My heart soared with joy at the thought of seeing and holding her in my arms again. I could not bring her to live in my uncle's house to share a room with four other men so, with the small amount of money I had managed to save, I rented a single room in New Kru Town and left my uncle's house.

The day that Josephine arrived, I was overjoyed. We were both electrified to see each other again. I took her home to our small, rented room. The place was bare. There was no bed, no chair, and no conveniences. We slept on the floor, ate on the floor, and stored our cooking pots on the floor. But nothing else mattered as long as we were together. I reached out to those in hiring positions at government offices and Josephine was able to get a job in the accounting department of the Ministry of Finance.

In July 2000, the second civil war broke out. I began to wonder why I had left Côte d'Ivoire for this uncertain life in Monrovia. We went for weeks with very little food. Many people in Monrovia died. In 2003, Charles Taylor was indicted by a UN-backed war crimes court for his alleged role in fueling Sierra Leone's 1991–2002 civil war. Later that year, warring factions signed a ceasefire, leading to talks to form a transitional government without Taylor. Nigerian soldiers arrived, as part of an African peacekeeping force, to be followed by a UN force. The government and rebels signed a peace deal, establishing a transitional administration to prepare for elections in 2005. An interim leader, Charles Gyude Bryant, a businessman and politician, was appointed chairman of the transitional government of Liberia in October 2003. His key role was to prepare the country for elections in October 2005. Rebel fighters also handed in their weapons under a UN-backed disarmament plan.

At the MOHSW, I rose from secretary to data clerk to data manager. The chief medical officer at that time, Dr. Nathaniel Bartee (now deceased), secured a three-month training course for me in malaria control and prevention, data management, and information technology in Ethiopia. When I returned home, I was assigned to the National Malaria Control Program (NMCP) as data manager. Dr. Benjamin Vonhm was then the program manager until 2001. He was succeeded by Dr. Joel J. Jones (now deceased), as program manager from 2002 to 2013. Dr. Jones and I worked together very closely. He was a good boss. Dr. Jones was a visionary who wanted to see malaria eliminated from Liberia and Africa in his lifetime. Unfortunately, he died on March 19, 2015. I was heartbroken.

While at NMCP, I was promoted several times to other positions—deputy program manager and acting program manager—each with more responsibilities. My income increased. Life became a little easier. I could see the possibilities of a brighter future, which I could not imagine without Josephine.

One day I told her to meet me after work. We met on Broad Street and walked into a jewelry store, where I said, "Pick any ring you want. I want to marry you."

She accepted my proposal, but she insisted that I ask her father for her hand.

I agreed; however, we wanted first to move to a better place, preferably an apartment outside of New Kru Town. Now that I was earning a decent salary and Josephine was also working, we could afford to live in a nicer place in a different neighborhood.

We took over Josephine's sister Annie's small single room in a rooming house in Sinkor, Old Road, on the other side of Monrovia. Annie had left Liberia for the United States in 2000 to join her husband, Victor, in Chicago, where he had immigrated in 1999. After settling into our new room, I took Josephine to visit her parents in Harper City to ask for her hand in marriage.

Mr. Kikeh did not seem surprised. After all, he had left his daughter in my care in Tabou for over a year, and I had taken care of her then. Mrs. Kikeh voiced her disapproval, but it didn't bother me because I knew I was not dirt poor anymore. I was in college, working a decent job, and earning a fair wage. Mr. Kikeh agreed to give me his daughter's hand, despite his wife's disapproval. On February 2, 2004, Josephine became my wife. Exactly a year later, on February 2, 2005, she gave birth to twin girls: Dehkontee and Nyennekon. In Kru, Dehkontee means "everything has time" and Nyennekon means "whatsoever you do you may be criticized."

A few months after the twins were born, we completed building our first home, which we started while living in New Kru town, with money we had saved. It was a small three-bedroom house in Gbankeh Town, Virginia, across the St. Paul River Bridge. As we settled in, we continued to save a portion of our salaries and put it toward building a bigger house in a better location. In Liberia it was rare that houses were sold. Most of the time, one had to construct a house from scratch. We first acquired the land, then laid down the foundation, and then set aside more funds to get the walls and roof up.

My life now was filled to the brim. I was married with two children, working full-time, and taking the maximum number of courses possible at the University of Liberia. I went to school in the evening after working all day, and I even registered for some classes on Saturdays. I attended the university from 1999 to 2005, and I graduated with my first degree, a Bachelor of Science in biology and chemistry. My intention had been to go on to medical school. However, medical school meant a substantial investment of time and money. I was already working full-time to support not only my own young family but my parents and siblings. Consequently, I chose law as a career, because I could go to law school late afternoons, when I left work, or during my lunch hour, and still maintain my position at the National Malaria Control Program (NMCP) as deputy program manager.

I attended the Louis Arthur Grimes School of Law at the University of Liberia from 2006 to 2009, earning a Bachelor of Law degree. As I climbed the ladder of academic success, I was promoted to positions with more responsibility at the MOHSW. Each position gave me more access to other opportunities and a pay raise, which enabled me to bring my brothers and sisters to Monrovia and help put them through school.

From 2004 to 2011, I was deputy program manager of NMCP. However, Dr. Jones went abroad on a study leave in 2007 to 2008, leaving me in charge as the acting program manager of NMCP, in addition to my role as his deputy. In this capacity, we secured the country's first malaria grant, in the amount of US$12 million, when then UN Secretary-General Kofi Annan established the Global Fund to accelerate the end of the AIDS, tuberculosis, and malaria epidemics. We were instrumental in changing the national drug policy for malaria from chloroquine to artemisinin-based combination therapy (ACT) and amodiaquine as first-line therapy. NMCP facilitated the treatment of over four million episodes of malaria and distributed more than five million mosquito nets to households around the country. We championed the "Hang Up, Keep Up" campaign, which provided at least three bed nets to every household. We were also instrumental in mobilizing another US$36 million for nationwide malaria programs, which resulted in a reduction in malaria prevalence from 66% to 28% in the span of five years.[4]

We did community household spraying with insecticides for mosquitos and developed the house-to-house strategy of every bed having one net. This is where I experienced real-time reporting and community mobilization. The malaria program and immunization programs helped develop my thinking on engaging the community, actually preparing me for the Ebola epidemic, in which I would adopt similar strategies and community-based initiatives.

Through the NMCP, we engineered bringing the President's Malaria Initiative (PMI) to Liberia, which became a PMI satellite country. According to the US CDC, "The U.S. President's Malaria Initiative (PMI) external icon is a U.S. Government initiative designed to drastically reduce malaria deaths and illnesses in target countries in sub-Saharan Africa with a long-term vision of a world without malaria. The initiative was announced on June 30, 2005, when President George W. Bush pledged to increase US funding of malaria prevention and treatment in sub-Saharan Africa by more than US$1.2 billion over five years (FY2006–FY2010)."[5] The President's Malaria Initiative (led by USAID and implemented with the CDC) delivers cost-effective, lifesaving interventions, alongside catalytic technical and operational assistance, with the goal of ending malaria. PMI has partnered with Liberia since 2008, helping to decrease child death rates by 18% through investments totaling almost US$159.8 million.[6]

During the same time period, I assisted in developing the National Tuberculosis Program and helped the HIV program introduce a single cross-border HIV/AIDS program, with funding support from the joint United Nations Programme on HIV/AIDS (UNAIDS). While working to minimize or eradicate infectious diseases, I championed awareness of the 1948 Universal Declaration of Human Rights (UDHR) so that Liberians throughout the country would know their rights, including rights for gender equity. The UDHR is defined as "a milestone document in the history of human rights." It was drafted by representatives with varying legal and cultural backgrounds from all regions of the world and was proclaimed by the United Nations General Assembly in Paris on

December 10, 1948 (General Assembly Resolution 217 A). This common standard of achievements for all peoples, and all nations, identifies for the first time fundamental human rights to be universally protected; it has been translated into more than 500 languages. The declaration is widely recognized as having inspired the permanent adoption of more than seventy human rights treaties at both the global and regional levels.[6]

Motorcycles were a primary means of transportation in Liberia. Working with the Ministry of Transportation, I advocated for a law mandating motorcycle riders wear helmets at all times to reduce casualties from accidents and lessen the public health toll of accidents, injuries, and fatalities.

Although I had earned a law degree, I loved my work and decided to dedicate my career to public health. This decision gave me the opportunity to be actively engaged in fostering the well-being of all Liberians. I was convinced that I had made the right choice when I was chosen by the government of Liberia in November 2009 to attend a three-week course in public health surveillance at Emory University in Atlanta, Georgia. Six months later, in mid-April 2010, my wife and I traveled to the United States for the very first time. Like many people, I had dreamed of coming to America. People in Liberia who had visited or studied in America often told me so many stories about this place. When they returned home, we called them "the been to." Now, I too was about to become a "been to."

We landed in Chicago to visit Josephine's sister, Annie, and her husband, Victor. Josephine was pregnant at the time, so I left her in Chicago and traveled to Atlanta two weeks later, arriving at Emory at the end of April. The course, Introduction to Public Health Surveillance, was organized by the CDC Surveillance, Epidemiology, and Laboratory Services and taught at the Hubert Department of Global Health, Emory University Rollins School of Public Health. I completed the course on schedule and returned to Chicago on May 17. Three days later, our son, Tolbert Jr., was born. I was elated to finally have a son. We returned to Liberia two weeks after Jr. was born.

Shortly after my return home, I resumed work at the Malaria Control Program as deputy program manager. My intention was to pursue a degree in public health at some point. In 2009, I had also applied to public health programs at three universities in the United States: Oklahoma State University, Harvard, and Johns Hopkins. I was accepted by all three institutions but had to defer because I could not afford the tuition and fees. So, I took the short course at Emory instead, which was fully funded by the government. In February 2011, I was awarded a full scholarship under a Global Fund Capacity Building grant to pursue a master's degree in public health. I chose to attend the Johns Hopkins Bloomberg School of Public Health in 2011, after two deferments due to funding constraints. For the first time in my life, my tuition and fees, plus accommodations and transportation costs, would be fully paid. Because I was on an approved work-related study-leave, the government of Liberia also continued to pay my salary (after six months, though, my salary was cut by half, in keeping with a civil service standing order). Because I had no worries about funding my education, I could rest assured that my family was provided for while I was away. I could simply go to school, focus on my studies, learn as much as I could, and enjoy the experience.

The program was rigorous, but being there changed the trajectory of my life. I studied public health and courses in epidemiology and biostatistics, health policy, international health, and public health and law. I stayed in the United States for eighteen months and did not go home until I graduated. It was difficult being away from Josephine and our three children. Every chance I got, I called to hear their voices and tell them how much I loved them. However, I knew this sacrifice of time and distance would pay off. I also earned three postgraduate certificates from Johns Hopkins in global public health, human rights, and epidemiology. After graduation, the Department of International Health at the Bloomberg School appointed me as an associate faculty member.

As I was preparing for the graduation ceremony on May 24, 2012, I received a phone call from my boss at the MOHSW, Dr. Bernice Dahn. She said that she considered recommending me for nomination as assistant minister for preventive services and deputy chief medical officer for prevention, replacing Mrs. Jesse Duncan, my immediate supervisor, who had been appointed as commissioner at the National AIDS Commission. I later found out that Mrs. Duncan had recommended me to the minister of health and Dr. Dahn to be her successor. Dr. Dahn said that Dr. Gwenigale subsequently recommended me to the president. I was elated! This meant that I would be going home to a higher-level post with more responsibilities and a salary increase. I believed Mrs. Duncan's recommendation was based on her time working with me when I was deputy and acting program manager at NMCP.

I was confirmed for my new role by the Senate in June 2012. This was a massive assignment. As we say in Liberia, it was a "big job"! I was now being referred to as the "honorable assistant minister of health," my first political appointment. God had promoted me once again, as my father often reminded me.

As head of the preventive services, I was in charge of more than twenty disease control programs headed by medical doctors, epidemiologists, and other public health experts. These included the National AIDS Control Program (NACP), National Malaria Control Program (NMCP), National Tuberculosis Control Program (NTBCP), the Expanded Programme on Immunization (EPI), and the divisions of mental health, noncommunicable diseases, and public health. My supervisory function focused on operational planning, strategic planning, and implementation of the maternal and child health program. Nutrition and social determinants of health (including environmental health, water sanitation, and hygiene) were also under my purview. My office continued advocating for policy change to reduce casualties from motorcycle injuries, working with the Ministry of Transportation and the police to make helmets mandatory for all motorcyclists and their passengers.

Motorcyclists (or "phen-phen boys," as they are called due to the excessive honking of their horns while in traffic) have a reputation of refusing to obey traffic rules. They often exceed the speed limit and move in and out of traffic without regard for other vehicles or drivers, often causing accidents with other vehicles and pedestrians. As a result, we restricted areas in the city center to motorcyclists, thereby significantly reducing the number of fatalities related to unsafe driving by phen-phen boys.

And now I had been asked to lead the IMS. In the quiet of my bedroom, I got down on my knees and prayed to God for guidance. I prayed for wisdom to identify and select the right people to fight in the war against Ebola.

When I spoke to Josephine about the role I would play and the magnitude of the task I had been given, she was dismayed! "With all the senior people in this government, why you?" she asked. "You see people dying, including trained medical doctors. Why you?" Entire families had been wiped away by Ebola, so my wife was right to be concerned.

The next morning, I called Dr. Kevin De Cock, who was advocating for the IMS, and Dr. Nestor Ndayimirije, the WHO resident representative in Liberia who advocated that the national coordination structure remain as it was under the minister. I wanted to consolidate my position and unveil my plans on how I envisioned the IMS would function. I asked for their guidance.

I chaired my first IMS meeting that day, August 14, in the MOHSW conference room on the fourth floor, informing all local and international partners that I, Tolbert G. Nyenswah, was now in charge of the national Ebola response.

CHAPTER 6

Security Challenge

Community Distrust and Resistance—West Point

Just before the Ebola incident management system (IMS) was created, a crisis erupted in a part of Monrovia called West Point. In early August 2014, the government imposed the isolation of Lofa County from the rest of the country, while the borders with Sierra Leone and Guinea had remained closed indefinitely since early July. West Point, a slum community near the sea, in central Monrovia, with population of roughly 50,000, and Dolo's Town, in Margibi County, with about 17,000 people[1] were later isolated. Certain communities in Lofa and Bomi Counties decided to impose their own self-isolation.

West Point is a densely populated beach slum. It has been the home of fishermen for decades. They live and raise their children by the sea and keep their canoes and motorboats close to their homes so they can conveniently cast nets at the crack of dawn for the catch of the day. This is how they make their living. This is how they care for their families and feed their children. This is their livelihood.

Rumors about Ebola abounded everywhere in Liberia, and West Point was no exception. Rumors persisted that Ebola was merely a myth, that it was not real, that the government was using Ebola to get money from the international community for personal use by corrupt government officials, including the president. Whether or not the rumors were true, people in the West Point community believed them. Young people living there, who were spreading the rumors, had a reputation for being rabble-rousers, streetwise, and defiant. Therefore, it was no surprise when Ebola virus disease (EVD) struck that West Point would indeed be a target—and not only for rumors and fabrications. West Point became a site of the EVD onslaught in every imaginable aspect.

There was no public hospital in West Point, although there was a health center called Star of the Sea, which was owned and operated by the Catholic Church, in addition to a few privately run community clinics and drug stores. According to Liberia's National Health Policy and Plan, a health center is the transition between primary and secondary levels of care and provides health services for twenty hours, with a maximum of forty inpatient beds and offering limited laboratory services. They are mandated to serve populations of 25,000 to 50,000. In contrast, public hospitals are expected to serve populations up to 250,000.[2] In July 2014, after a few residents in the community began to show signs and symptoms of Ebola, fear gripped the community. Several households became infected. Dead bodies were thrown into the streets, and sick people were left in the streets to die.

Because of the population density in West Point, the government of Liberia made a strategic decision to quarantine the entire community for twenty-one days, the full length of the Ebola virus incubation period. There was community resistance to this form of isolation, so a compromise was reached. By late July, the ministry identified a school building in West Point that could be used as a temporary isolation unit, to move sick people from their homes and off the streets. This would prevent secondary infections of EVD. The ministry assured the community that this building would only be used to quarantine people who actually lived in West Point. The MOHSW would supply food, water, mattresses, and other supplies to make the school an acceptable environment as a temporary isolation facility. Health care workers and a team of active case finders were deployed to the isolation site.

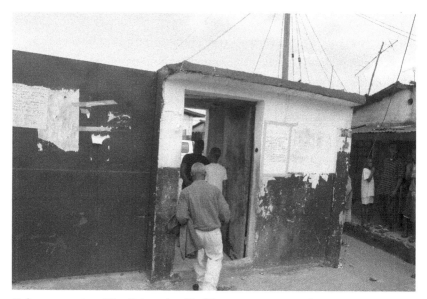
Only entrance into West Point school building—temporary isolation unit

At first, the procedures seemed to be working. The residents were adjusting to or tolerating their restrictive situation. Subsequently, news spread to other communities in and around Monrovia that West Point had a designated isolation or Ebola treatment unit (ETU). After the rumors surfaced, West Pointers saw their community swarmed by government-owned and operated ambulances, private pickup trucks, taxis, and even wheelbarrows that carried huge numbers of suspected Ebola patients from other communities.

The West Point community was infuriated. They said that the government had deceived them and taken them for fools. They no longer trusted the government; in their eyes, the agreement had been violated. Expressing their anger, young agitators took to the streets. They stormed into the temporary isolation unit in the school building and looted all the supplies and equipment that the government had delivered a few days prior.

President Sirleaf was informed of the community's reaction and distress. She convened a meeting at her office, where some cabinet officials suggested that the government introduce a curfew and elevate the quarantine of West Point. What they did not seem to realize was that those decisions would not help to stop Ebola from spreading there.

Meanwhile, Dolo's Town, another densely populated slum outside of the capital in Margibi County, approximately nine miles from the Roberts International Airport, had reported an increasing number of suspected EVD cases and Ebola-related deaths. The case fatality rate had significantly increased in a short span of time. At the meeting, officials suggested that the government quarantine Dolo's Town, like they did West Point, and impose a strict curfew. Dolo's Town's population was much smaller than West Point's, and the town was far removed from the fanfare that now surrounded West Point. We did not expect the impact would be the same. When it did surface, community resistance was minimal compared to the fracas in West Point.

At the time, Chief Medical Officer Dr. Bernice Dahn was running the national Ebola response. In one of our technical group meetings at the MOHSW, when Minister of Health Dr. Walter Gwenigale was away at a task force meeting, Dr. Dahn allowed me to voice my concerns. I mentioned that it was counterproductive to take extreme measures and subject young people to undue hardship when they were already trying to protect themselves from a horrifying disease, while watching their friends and relatives die in rapid succession. I felt that heightened restrictions in West Point would further exacerbate the already volatile situation we had encountered. People distrusted the government. Some even believed that they would be injected with Ebola and later die a horrible death. I warned that we would only be able to control Ebola transmission by working in concert with the affected communities. If we quarantined our citizens, we would have to provide them with food and water. I suggested that we focus on traditional public health measures, such as active case finding and contact tracing (which involved doing household interviews and searches to actively trace those who had come in contact with an infected or suspected case) and implementing safe burial practices by setting up a team to collect bodies, properly prepare them, and safely and respectful bury the dead. I proposed that cases be managed appropriately based on signs and symptoms, and by setting up isolation units and building ETUs, with a capacity to admit and treat or provide supportive care. Perhaps if the government had taken these actions, the crisis that followed might have been avoided. But the president and her national security council decided to quarantine West Point and impose a curfew. Acting upon the president's directives, riot police and soldiers moved into West Point with tanks, scrap wood, and barbed wire to seal off 50,000—mostly young and energetic—people inside a slum, believing they could contain the Ebola outbreak in Liberia this way.

Naturally, residents became more infuriated. They felt they were being blamed for spreading a disease they were still trying to understand. They believed the government had lied to them about the temporary isolation facility in their community, which should have been for them alone. They felt the government failed to quickly collect the dead bodies from the streets and left them to deal with the stench and sight of decaying flesh. Their agitation intensified. Hundreds of residents in West Point clashed with the military and police. Gunfire erupted. A

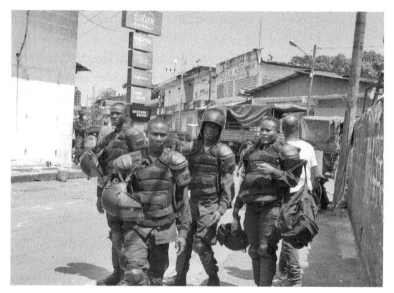

Liberian National Police Riot Squad entering West Point

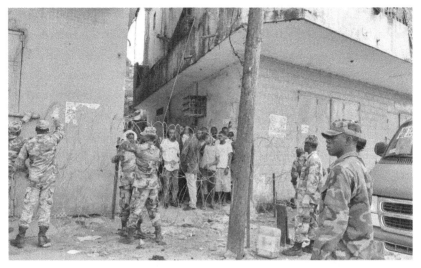

Liberian military barricading West Point residents behind barbed wire

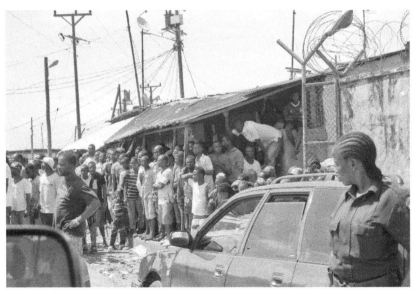

West Point residents forced behind barricade

sixteen-year-old, Shacki Kamara, was fatally shot while trying to cross the barbed wire, as security forces fired into the air incessantly to disperse the crowd. The quarantine morphed into a nightmare. Tensions between the community and the government increased as residents remained defiant, despite being forcefully kept behind barbed wire fences and makeshift gates, guarded by rifle-toting, trigger-happy riot police and the military.

On August 19, President Sirleaf addressed the nation: "We have been unable to control the spread due to continued denials, cultural burying practices, disregard for the advice of health workers, and disrespect for the warnings by the government. . . . Fellow citizens, these measures are meant to save lives."[3] The following day, she imposed a nationwide nighttime curfew, from 6 p.m. to 6 a.m., in addition to the existing quarantine isolating West Point and Dolo's Town. She ordered all movie theaters, nightclubs, and other gathering places closed; stopped ferry service to the peninsula around West Point; and dispatched the Liberian National Coast Guard to patrol the surrounding waters.

Police moved swiftly to seal off the peninsula. Angry crowds assembled, becoming violent when a local government representative returned to her home in West Point to get her family out. Hundreds surrounded her house until security forces packed the family into a car, fired into the air, and hustled them away.

At the incident management system emergency meeting that day, some officials with deep-rooted ties to the local community, having grown up there or who still had relatives there, spoke up. They raised the point that the government's response to communal resistance to a public health intervention was overwhelmingly aggressive at a time in our history when we were besieged by a plague, when people lived with fear and desperation of the unknown, as whole families dropped dead suddenly, right before their eyes. Certainly, a less invasive approach would have been advisable if the intervention was to be accepted. Perhaps prior conversations with community leaders, addressing concerns and constraints, would have better prepared the community for the intervention. It was noted that even if community residents resisted the

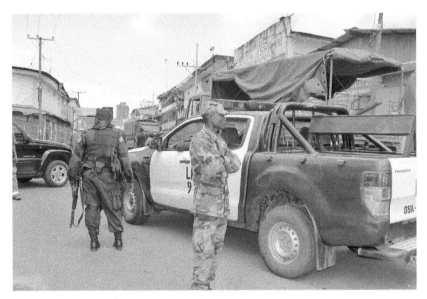

Liberian National Police and military sealing off West Point peninsula

government's plans, their respect for their leaders was resolute and therefore they would have complied with what their leaders requested. Military force would not have been necessary. The IMS recognized that the cooperation of local leaders was integral to arresting the epidemic; they were the bridge between the government and the community that held them in high regard. A meeting with community leaders was arranged. The general consensus was that blanket quarantine of a community with military force and police violence is not the appropriate response to community resistance to any public health intervention, anywhere in the world, especially not in resource-constrained environments where poverty, poor sanitation, and infrastructural challenges may be impediments to compliance.

The use of force to quarantine these communities was a serious error. Initial community involvement and ownership would have helped greatly. Community-based initiatives were mitigating factors in Ebola outbreaks reported in other areas. This approach, which should have been employed earlier, would eventually prove crucial in curtailing the epidemic.

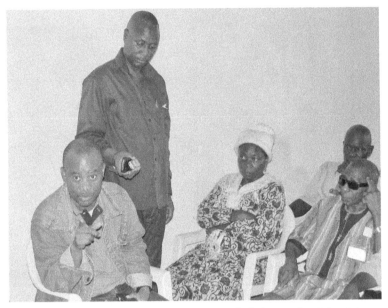

Labor minister and human rights lawyer Kofi Woods (*left, seated*) at West Point community meeting. Woods grew up in West Point.

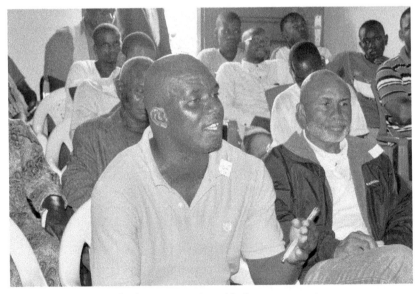

West Point community leaders at a meeting with the government

On August 30, the president lifted the quarantines. This brought some relief to the people of West Point. But the end of Ebola was nowhere in sight.

When I became the incident manager, on August 14, 2014, I began creating a plan and putting together a core team of professionals and experts. I set out to identify and catalog what human, technical, financial, and logistical resources were actually available, and to determine how these resources would be managed for specified response objectives in the interest of public health and scientific understanding.

The US CDC committed to assisting the MOHSW in developing the IMS. To achieve this, the CDC insisted that certain structures be put in place. There had to be better implementation of feedback regarding daily tasks and ways to determine whether or not they were completed. Planning could not be ad hoc like it had been with the task force—planning had to look at long-term processes that would unfold over a period of months, perhaps even years.

All fifteen counties had to be active in national response activities and given more appropriate guidance in outlining individual county response priorities. County operations had to be supported based on both their own and national priorities.

Disaster and emergency management experts were to be given priority in recruitment. The MOHSW had to consider setting up a formal Emergency Operations Center (EOC) as a central point to handle incoming information and requests. The IMS was expected to share all pertinent information daily with a higher-level, inter-ministerial Ebola Task Force, which was chaired by the president and the minister of internal affairs.

The inauguration of the IMS was challenging. We were operating under a new structure while dealing with evolving policies, responding to new situations, and overseeing the implementation of key response activities. The first phase of the epidemic had been hampered by weak decision-making and insufficient attention to logic, in part because of the existing hierarchical leadership approach. This contributed to amplification of the epidemic. Now, a distributed leadership approach replaced the old hierarchies. In addition to sharing leadership responsibility and authority, the distributed leadership approach involved strategic engagement with stakeholders and intensive communication.

The CDC's recommendations began to yield greater efficiency. Task force meetings were significantly reorganized to allow attendance by only one member of essential response committees authorized to make decisions on the committee's behalf. Obstacles to implementing decisions made the day before were identified and discussed. The new IMS included input and meeting participation by key international partners. The response structure represented the principal sources of data for describing the epidemic.

Alongside Dr. Kevin De Cock, the CDC's team lead, was Edward N. Rouse, who served as the CDC's logistics section chief. Ed Rouse was helpful to me in understanding my position, terms of reference, and the IMS organizational structure as a whole. Once I was equipped with the information, I started to reshape positions, redeploy staff, and bring in new people.

To improve coordination of county operations with the national response priorities, I selected Dr. Francis Kateh as deputy incident manager. At the time Dr. Kateh was the medical director of the Tappita Hospital in Nimba County and had been assigned to help with the Ebola response in Margibi.

We established a unit that provided support for financial, administrative, planning, and logistical matters. Miatta Gbanya was appointed deputy for finance and administration. Before the advent of Ebola, the MOHSW had a designated account, into which donors such as UNICEF, the UK's Department for International Development (DFID), Irish Aid, and the French government, agreed to put money for programs implemented by the ministry. This was known as the MOHSW Health Sector Pool Fund, which was managed by the Jacob Hughes Foundation. Ms. Gbanya worked for the Hughes Foundation as manager of this pool fund and had the reputation of being efficient in executing her responsibilities. With this in mind, I purposely asked the minister to allow Ms. Gbanya to assist with IMS administration, finance, and payrolls for response workers because I believed she would be rigorous with payroll management and timely payment of response workers. Ms. Gbanya is also a nurse who worked in public health. During the crisis, she visited ETUs on occasion.

As the incident manager, I reported directly to President Sirleaf daily and communicated with her at several other intervals during the course of the day as well, to keep her abreast of events as they unfolded. In addition, I briefed CMO Dahn and Minister Gwenigale as often as possible on events. This did not sit well with my superiors or my fellow junior colleagues at the MOHSW.

IMS History and Structure

The concept of the command-and-control structure of an incident management system originated in the 1970s, in an attempt by the US Forest Service to coordinate responses to California's frequent and unpredictable wildfires. In 1987, the IMS structure was endorsed by the US Federal Emergency Management Agency (FEMA) and subsequently by the US Coast Guard, in 1989. In the aftermath of the September 11, 2001, terrorist attacks, the incident management system became the national model for the coordination of emergency response adopted by US Department of Homeland Security; subsequently, the approach was recognized internationally, as well.[4]

Liberia's IMS had a command staff, as well as operations, logistical, and financial support structures. The IMS had key technical committees, also called thematic areas or pillars, for epidemiological surveillance, contact tracing, case management, dead body management, laboratory, logistics and support system, communications / community engagement / social mobilization, county operations, nutrition, and psychosocial support. Each area was headed by a designated senior staff member from within the MOHSW and other government agencies. Because the response was just not for health, the IMS staff included trained logisticians and information and communication technology (ICT) specialists, all of whom reported directly to me, the incident manager, in daily morning briefings and throughout the day as was necessary. The IMS reported twice weekly to the national consultative group, the Presidential Advisory Council on Ebola (PACE), chaired by the president of Liberia and cochaired by the speaker of the House of Representatives. As the incident manager, I presented these reports in person. Separate from the technically focused IMS, the PACE acted as a think tank, bringing policy issues and information to the president, such as cremation, reopening of schools, curfews, Ebola vaccine trials, border closings, and travel restrictions.

The IMS provided the opportunity for essential international partners to more fully participate and give their input based on their technical expertise. The concept of "one team, one leader, one operational plan and one strategy" was adopted. This change in strategy based on prevailing Ebola caseloads led to rapid isolation and treatment of Ebola (known as the RITE strategy), which was prominent in identifying Ebola cases in rural communities and other hard-to-reach areas.

Between August and December 2014, the IMS held close to 150 daily meetings. Thematic groups had separate site meetings in the temporary EOC on 18th Street, in the Sinkor area of Monrovia.

There were two kinds of meetings held each day: operational meetings from 8 to 8:45 a.m. and technical meetings from 9 to 10 a.m. Depending on the agenda, the meetings would sometimes extend thirty minutes or more. On Fridays, the IMS held open meetings with nongovernmental organizations (NGOs) and other civil society organizations. Country representatives from crucial external partners also participated in these IMS meetings, including WHO, CDC, African Union, certain UN agencies, and USAID, which activated its Disaster Assistance Response Team (DART) under the Office of Foreign Disaster Assistance (OFDA).

We introduced the *One Plan, One Strategy, One Response* slogan, aimed at organizations and individuals who descended upon Liberia, attempting to duplicate the government's official response efforts. For their own purpose, they took action and independently solicited funding in the name Liberia, without discussing or coordinating their plans with the government. These entities knowingly and selfishly intended to undermine Liberia's Ebola response funding streams and programmatic activities by taking advantage of our disastrous situation with the sole intention of enriching themselves. Ebola became a fair game, a get-rich-quick scheme. Organizations that never existed previously anywhere in the world suddenly emerged on the scene, claiming to have expertise to contribute to the response in one way or another, only to later be found out not to have any expertise at all. There was a lot of deception and lack of transparency. Ebola became a breeding ground for greedy and unskilled foreigners. The sad thing is, many managed to infiltrate the system and reap a fortune.

Decentralizing the Incident Management System at the County Level

When the national IMS was organized, the health system was already fragile. The county system was even more delicate. To partially deal with this situation, we appointed county-level incident managers and formed technical committees with specific goals. The purpose of the decentralization was to streamline the national response framework implemented by the MOHSW, establish a clear chain of command, ensure accountability, improve efficiency, assist with identifying gaps, and permit a national-level public health response in each of the fifteen counties. Before the decentralization activities began, we identified critical county-level functions. Each county had to identify the personnel who would be responsible for conducting its response. The number of cases in the county had to be determined. Contact tracing mechanisms had to be in place. Worker safety considerations had to be addressed, with assurances that personal protective equipment received from the ministry would be immediately distributed to health facilities in the county. A mechanism for transmitting to and receiving information from national headquarters had to be established.

Emergency operations centers with designated incident managers were set up in all fifteen counties. In some counties, however, these incident managers were county health officers (CHOs). If the CHO was not performing as expected in implementing response activities, they were replaced by another incident manager, who was not a county health official. This replacement did not affect the CHO's position as a MOHSW-assigned official.

To maintain focus and accountability, each committee had one person designated as the lead, responsible for coordinating the team, as well as presenting and assigning members with tasks identified by the incident manager for a given twenty-four-hour operational period. Team members reported only to the lead and were expected to conduct and complete their tasks throughout the twenty-four-hour operational period, especially while the team lead was attending the daily 9 a.m. meetings.

Meetings and staffing needs varied depending on the role and goal of the technical committee—some committees had significantly greater staffing needs due to subdivisions within the committee. For example, the case management team included a member who reported on activities and gaps for each of its subdivisions or units (treatment, ambulance, burial, psychosocial, and worker safety units). We included the psychosocial unit under case management to improve efficiency of the 9 a.m. meeting. The worker safety unit was responsible for conducting needs assessments for personal protective equipment. This unit also worked with social mobilization and communications to ensure that public health messaging was appropriate. Social mobilization handled messaging for the general public and communications informed stakeholders, partners, and the international community.

Each team was restricted to five members. Team members were expected to anticipate specific needs for the following twenty-four-hour operational period, based on discussions and information collected from a particular county. On the national level, committee members were expected to carry out specific objectives and priorities identified by the IMS through interaction with county officials. During the initial period, operational support based on a specified need was given to Montserrado County, which had the largest population and caseload. Operational support was subsequently provided to the remaining counties in Liberia.

I was exceptionally pleased with the way the IMS was established and run. It is worth noting that an IMS can work well when it is decentralized. We organized specific county-level incident management systems to handle the surge of Ebola cases in urban areas like Monrovia, with its population of 1.5 million. Each county-level IMS reported to the central IMS, through Thomas Nagbe, who was the designated IMS county coordinator already employed at the central MOH. The Montserrado County IMS and other IMSs across the country set up their own thematic areas patterned after the central IMS. These units functioned with both national and international technical partners that supported them at the county level. Technically, each county took charge of its own response. However, the national IMS in Monrovia was responsible for all major decisions on the response. The beauty of this was that, with good coordination, response efforts became much more effective. When it was more difficult to control the outbreak in a county, as was the case in Lofa and Grand Cape Mount Counties, the national IMS moved in with officials from international agencies to provide technical, logistical, moral, and financial support. Dr. Anthony Banbury, special representative of the UN secretary-general, who headed the first-ever UN Mission for Ebola Emergency Response (UNMEER), along with Dr. David Nabarro, head of the UN Ebola Response, and Dr. Bruce Aylward, assistant director-general of WHO, responsible for the Ebola response, visited Grand Cape Mount County (western region of Liberia), where we held an IMS strategy meeting. Dr. Aylward also served as the secretary-general's special envoy on Ebola, to provide strategic and policy direction for an enhanced international response and galvanize essential support for affected communities and countries.[5] His presence with Dr. Nabarro and other high-ranking international civil servants at this meeting in the western region, where the outbreak was spiraling out of control, was a game changer.

Coordination of Response Activities

Under the directive of President Sirleaf, the MOHSW was to lead the incident management system and provide overall management of the national Ebola response. This major role was not to be deferred to any foreign entity. The strategic plan outlined levels of authority, organizational relationships, and descriptions of specific programs and tasks to be undertaken by the IMS exclusively, in coordination with the government's line ministries or with selective international partner agencies. The IMS was to serve as the foundation for the government's planning and response support for the Ebola outbreak. The overall objective of the IMS was to stop Ebola transmission and avert secondary consequences.

The IMS provided an efficient national response. First and foremost, improvement in command and control was noteworthy. Second, the technical team structure with defined prerequisites for each team greatly facilitated efficiency in response goals. Third, identifying mechanisms to achieve these prerequisites made achievement more likely. Fourth, streamlining and transmitting data throughout national, county, and district levels and to key collaborators facilitated overall coordination.

The basis of EVD control required active case finding, isolation of active cases, providing medical care to active cases, documenting and follow-up on primary and secondary contacts, and isolation of contacts who became ill. If a contact remained well twenty-one days postexposure, that person was discharged from further follow-up. The incubation of the Ebola virus spans two to twenty-one days, even though most exposed contacts, if infected, manifest symptoms within eight to ten days after exposure.[6]

The IMS priorities on Ebola control interventions were mainly focused on surveillance and contact tracing; laboratory and case testing; infection prevent and control; establishing Ebola treatment units; safe and dignified burials, taking into account religious affiliation, culture, and tradition; and social mobilization and community engagement.

The IMS placed emphasis on conducting daily response activities within each twenty-four-hour operational period, replicating key IMS-associated activities and functions in each county, providing technical assistance by deploying local and international staff to work with county teams, and decentralizing the response process to halt transmission of the EVD.

As the national incident manager, I led a team to conduct several field visits to all fifteen counties to assess selected areas and identify suitable sites for the construction of ETUs. We also visited burial sites and existing ETUs, either to check on the operations or discharge procedures for survivors from ETUs across Liberia. I supported and attended regional meetings with Guinea and Sierra Leone.

As the CDC team had noted in its recommendations of August 1, "For a public health response to be effective, it is critical that there be well-defined roles and responsibilities; a clear chain of command; and enforcement of accountability."[7]

On the other side of the African continent, in the Democratic Republic of the Congo (DRC), security challenges that plagued Liberia's response repeated itself in the tenth and eleventh Ebola outbreaks in the DRC in 2019–21, three to six years later, this time at a very alarming rate. On October 8, 2021, the Ministry of Health announced that a new laboratory-confirmed case of Ebola virus disease (EVD) had been detected in Butsili Health Area, Beni Health Zone in North Kivu Province. Earlier, an EVD outbreak affected North Kivu Province, which was declared over on May 3, 2021, according to the WHO. A 3-year-old male in early October developed symptoms including physical weakness, loss of appetite, abdominal pain, breathing difficulty, dark stool, and blood in his vomit, typical signs of EVD. He died on October 6. The following day, samples were tested at the National Institute of Biomedical Research (INRB) laboratory in Beni for molecular analysis. These were later sent to the Rodolphe Mérieux INRB Laboratory, Goma on October 8 and EVD was confirmed by reverse transcription polymerase chain reaction (RT-PCR) on the same day.[8]

The DRC's national Ebola response was hindered by conflicts between the government and rebel forces, which resulted in violence and more disputes. Dr. Richard Valery Mouzoko Kiboung, a Cameroonian epidemiologist working with WHO on the Ebola response, was killed on April 19, 2019, when rebels attacked the Butembo hospital in the eastern region of the DRC, which had become an Ebola epicenter.[9] WHO suspended its work in the DRC following Dr. Kiboung's killing. Understandably, other international response workers were overcome by fear and frustration. Addressing the senseless murder of his staff, Dr. Tedros Adhanom Ghebreyesus, director of the WHO, tweeted, "Today we lost one of our very own: Dr Richard Valery Mouzoko Kiboung, an epidemiologist deployed in the Ebola response in DRC, during a hospital attack in Butembo. We grieve together with his family during this difficult time."[9] Being persistent, persuasive, and by engaging the communities to own and participate, rather than deny and resist, significantly impacted the response and turned the epidemic around in Liberia.[10]

CHAPTER 7

Interventions

What We Did and How We Did It

Following the establishment of the incident management system (IMS), and with international support finally forthcoming, Liberia began to gain control of the crisis. Several crucial interventions were implemented as we began receiving financial and technical assistance from outside the country. (See chapter 8 for a closer look at the role of international partners.)

Contact Tracing

Contact tracing and active case finding were key strategies that ended the 2014–2016 Ebola outbreak in West Africa.[1] Contact tracing is an essential public health tool that is used every day to stop disease transmission, such as for tuberculosis, syphilis, and HIV.[1] WHO described contact tracing as "a process of identifying, assessing, and managing people who have been exposed to a disease to prevent onward transmission."[2] During the Ebola epidemic, we tracked all persons who had direct contact with an Ebola-infected individual or dead body and monitored them for the twenty-one-day incubation period, from the time of their last contact with the infected source. Ebola incubation ranges from two to twenty-one days after exposure, when symptoms

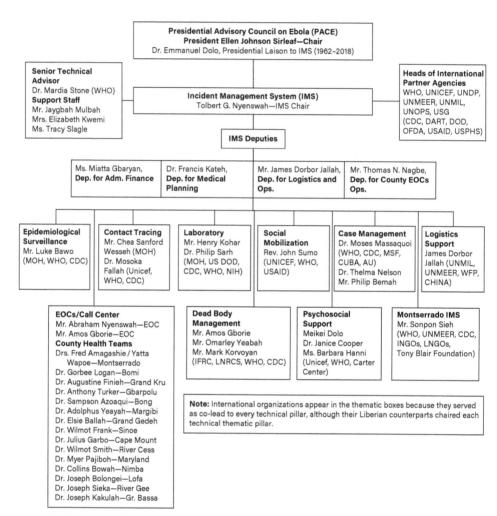

IMS Structure Diagram. Incident Management System / Ebola Virus Disease Response Structure: Liberia (2014–2016). Courtesy of Tolbert Nyenswah

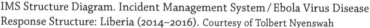

could manifest. On average, most people get sick within eight to ten days after exposure.[1] Contact tracing is especially useful in averting severe disease in high-risk individuals by making them aware of their exposure so that they seek medical care quickly if they do develop symptoms.

Through contact tracing, we were able to readily identify contacts who were beginning to manifest symptoms of Ebola and quickly isolated them in Ebola treatment units (ETUs) or, in some instances, in their homes, followed by daily monitoring visits by at least two members of the contact tracing team. Whenever the home was unsuitable for isolation, we rented small houses or apartments, which were used as temporary isolation units because there were no isolation facilities in most areas. People who had been in contact with the same infected person were isolated in the same house or apartment. Contacts from the same community or same environment, such as a health facility, were similarly grouped. The daily onslaught of excessive caseloads, reported nationally, hindered our efforts at active case finding and contact tracing. In Monrovia and surrounding counties, it seemed like there was no end in sight. However, in rural counties far removed from Monrovia and Lofa, there were significantly fewer cases. In these areas, social and community mobilization strategies were utilized to promote awareness, while simultaneously engaging and educating communities. Halting the epidemic in more populous areas (Lofa and Montserrado Counties) warranted more rigorous case finding and contact tracing methods. We also needed to recruit and deploy more contact tracers in the field. Ultimately, we had a team of roughly 10,000 contact tracers nationwide, 4,000 of whom were assigned to Monrovia.[3,4]

In southeastern Liberia, cases were at a minimum, with Grand Gedeh County reporting fewer than five cases.[3] By January 2015, two-thirds of all counties did not have a confirmed case or contact under follow-up. On average, the number of contacts per case was estimated at five.[3,4] The percentage of contacts traced daily was roughly 92%.[3,4] Contacts that manifested symptoms of Ebola and were initially reported as cases by contact tracers were estimated at 6% in eight counties.[3,4]

A rigorous contact tracing and active case finding system, headed by the assistant minister of health for vital statistics, Hon. C. Stanford Wesseh, was buttressed through the community-based initiative (CBI), headed by Dr. Mosoka Fallah and funded by the United Nations Development Programme (UNDP). What had been advocated during the initial phase of the response was now coming to fruition. The community-based program was fully recognized by the IMS, enabling IMS members with ties to local communities to better understand that less-invasive Ebola control interventions were more likely to be accepted.[5] CBI altered the dynamics in disease transmission by bringing certain cultural details to the government's attention. Before the emergence of the CBI, tradition, cultural sensitivity, and infrastructural constraints were not taken into account when the government made policy decisions, when public health messages were crafted, or when interventions were planned or implemented. Community leaders were never a part of the process, resulting in community distrust and resistance to the interventions.

CBI became more significant after the West Point fiasco. Volunteers were recruited from within communities and trained to coordinate surveillance activities in districts infested with active Ebola cases. Affected districts were identified by coordinators from the MOHSW, who then organized an open meeting for community, tribal, and religious leaders, along with other stakeholders in the district, to get a sense of their perceptions about the government's handling of the Ebola response. Participants were expected to give honest opinions, highlighting what worked, pointing out what was flawed, and suggesting alternatives to improve response activities, specific to their respective communities.

On September 17, a district-wide pilot program promoting awareness of Ebola was launched, with guidance from international public health advisors.[5] The goal was to encourage community engagement in the response. A local team comprised of members from within the districts was assigned to map the area to assess human resource requirements. Community leaders who attended the initial meeting recruited community members for a one-day training session on active surveillance. Each CBI volunteer was then assigned approximately twenty-five households to survey daily.[5] The CBI volunteers received daily sustenance allowances as a token of appreciation for their diligent work. Supervisors and other members received funding as well, from the UNDP. The UNDP also provided funding for CBI training. A total of 6,500 trainees were hired as community coordinators. They were given appropriate tools and equipped for six months; each person was paid roughly US$65 per month.[5] At the training session, county-level CBI coordinators reviewed data collection forms with community members. Supervisors received and were trained to use mobile telephones, preloaded with a user-friendly application for submitting data in real time. This data informed case investigation, contact tracing, burial, and ambulance teams to rapidly respond to incidents. Using the forms, trained community members made daily reports on the sick, deceased, visitors, and other factors that influenced Ebola transmission in their communities. Hierarchical reporting and coordinating structures were established, with community surveillance coordinators submitting these forms to their immediate supervisors, who sent aggregate data to the district-level supervisors. The CBI program was a very effective means of contact tracing and active case finding. Unfortunately, its implementation began rather late in the outbreak.

Case Management and Ebola Treatment Units

ETUs designed specifically for isolating and treating patients with Ebola virus disease had been set up in other places with prior EVD outbreaks. Because EVD has usually emerged in rural areas of countries considered to be underdeveloped, ETUs were usually set up by international humanitarian agencies or nongovernmental organizations (NGOs). They would bring specialized staff and equipment, including premium personal protective equipment, essential in preventing staff from contracting the disease while working in an ETU. Médecins Sans Frontières (MSF) had set up ETUs in several countries, run mainly by international health professionals with support from local employees. MSF had a reputation of providing high-quality care in ETUs (e.g., intravenous fluids, treatment of co-infections, and other supportive care). However, mechanical ventilation is not used and laboratory investigations are not conducted in the ETU. Working in an ETU is no easy feat. Conditions are intense and staff have to wear restrictive PPEs at all times, which are often very hot and uncomfortable. They have to be put on in a certain way and removed in a particular way to prevent staff contamination, especially after tending to an EVD patient. A separate section within the facility, suitable to safely decontaminate PPEs, is critical. So is an appropriate waste disposal system and procedures for safe removal of corpses to be taken to safe burial sites. The high-quality, twenty-four-hour care provided by MSF in ETUs required "10 or more health care staff per EVD patient, including physicians, nurses, hygienists, cleaners, and ancillary support staff."[6]

In mid-July, Liberia had only two 20-bed ETUs: one in Foya, Lofa County, the first epicenter, and the other at ELWA Hospital in Monrovia. At that time, Samaritan's Purse, the US-based NGO, operated and provided trained expatriate and local staff at both ETUs. Their staff had also been trained by MSF, which was working concurrently on the Ebola outbreak response in Guinea and Sierra Leone.[6] By late July, Samaritan's Purse withdrew its international staff from Liberia after three health care workers (two Americans and one Liberian) became infected with the Ebola virus in the ETU at ELWA Hospital. As the number of cases escalated, ETU staff, then primarily MOHSW staff, were inundated. They did not have the capacity and could barely continue to function. Both ETUs were overloaded with EVD cases. In July and early August, it was burdensome finding ways to isolate EVD patients in their respective counties, because isolation units simply did not exist throughout the country. Even in Monrovia, isolation was a challenge. With limited bed space, when patients flocked to ELWA in huge numbers, they had to hang around the grounds outside, on the grass, in wheelbarrows, on blankets, in taxis or however they got there, waiting for admission.

As cases increased, we had no isolation units in most counties and needed many more isolation facilities in Monrovia. Our predicament was that we did not have the necessary infrastructure, human capacity, or financial resources to handle the epidemic. We needed every kind of basic supply—everything: chlorine, surgical gloves, body bags—and better capacity to handle corpses. We didn't have the resources, and the international humanitarian assistance we expected was not forthcoming. It was a struggle. According to a February 2016 review of the MSF's communications and advocacy in the Ebola response from March 2014 through March 2015, "WHO was reluctant to interact with MSF at a high level. MSF's critique of WHO resulted in lack of trust from their side. MSF's interaction with institutional bodies was mainly handled by the Ebola specialist, but on reflection, engagement from a more senior representative at an earlier stage may have been helpful. Engaging with regional health actors or [WHO Regional Office for Africa] was not seen as a priority by MSF."[6]

MOHSW surveillance data from mid-August showed that only 25% of all reported EVD patients at the time had been admitted to ETUs.[7] We believed this was underreported. Furthermore, the high case fatality rate in the Montserrado ETU, possibly the result of inadequate staffing, suggested that the treatment units were providing little clinical benefit. As a result, the Liberia Medical and Dental Council (LMDC), the licensing umbrella of the medical professionals in Liberia, then headed by Dr. John Mulbah (an obstetrician-gynecologist), changed the treatment regimen and case management protocol. The head of the IMS case management pillar, Dr. Moses Massaqoui, also drew up new clinical guidelines for treating Ebola patients. Because of the high case fatality rates, the IMS endorsed a new treatment protocol for all ETUs in the country, which included administering IV fluids. We discovered that an ETU that was not properly managed may have been more dangerous to patients and staff than lower levels of care.

Nationally, the total bed capacity was up to 650 (with the potential to quickly open 1,219 beds)[8] across fourteen ETUs within seven of the fifteen counties by September 2014: Montserrado (6), Bomi (1), Nimba (1), Bong (1), Margibi (3), Lofa (1), and Grand Gedeh (1).[8] An ETU (Monrovia Medical Unit) was set up in Margibi County, close to Roberts International Airport, specifically to care for health care workers infected with Ebola. The US government opened the Monrovia Medical Unit on November 25, 2014.[9] The twenty-five-bed field hospital was built by the US Department of Defense and was staffed by US Public Health Service clinicians. It was one component of a broader effort to protect international and Liberian health care workers who courageously volunteered to treat Ebola patients in Liberia.[9] Each ETU would start at ten beds and scale up to more beds as necessary. Some ETUs served as training sites only. The goal was to establish seventeen ETUs nationwide by the end of October 2014, with a total of 2,100 beds in all facilities combined.[8]

As of February 9, 2014, Liberia reported 8,864 Ebola cases, of which 3,147 were laboratory confirmed.[10] Most of these cases were from rural areas. It was believed that Monrovia was fueling the outbreak to remote areas, when infected persons left Monrovia for their rural villages and towns. This was of concern to the IMS. Consequently, in August 2014, the Ministry of Health and Social Welfare team, led by Dr. Francis Kateh, IMS deputy for medical planning, began systematically investigating and responding to Ebola outbreaks in remote areas, supported by the World Health Organization, the CDC, and others. Many of these areas lacked mobile telephone service, easy road access, or basic infrastructure. Therefore, interventions had to be flexible and targeted.[10] Development of a national strategy for rapid isolation and treatment of Ebola (RITE) began in early October.[10] This strategy focused on enhancing capacity of county health teams (CHTs) to investigate outbreaks in remote areas and lead tailored responses through effective and efficient coordination of technical and operational assistance, from the MOHSW central level and international partners.[10] Setting up community care centers (CCCs) in each county was another component of the RITE strategy. These CCCs were connected to county health facilities in hotspots where rapid isolation was crucial.

Nutritional support was essential for patients in treatment units and care centers. Patients already malnourished before contracting Ebola seemed to die more quickly. We observed that poor nutrition resulted in much higher death rates in some treatment units. Ebola and severe nutritional deficiencies compromise a patient's immune system and immune response to fight off disease. In order to address these vulnerabilities, we needed a well-balanced meal plan for our patients and a dedicated nutrition team. Nadu Cooper, a retired WHO professional, was contracted to put together the team. In her wisdom, she subcontracted female restaurateurs across the country to provide catering services for the ETUs and CCCs. These restaurateurs constituted the Nutrition pillar of the Ebola response. They were divided into small, county-specific teams, each of which provided three nutritionally balanced meals per day for each patient, which complemented clinical EVD protocols based on a patient's clinical signs and symptoms. Nutrition teams had to adhere to strict infection prevention and control (IPC) standards. Mrs. Cooper determined the kinds of foods (including local dishes and coconut water) and other culinary commodities that were necessary to safely prepare the patients' meals. Teams were appropriately managed regarding handling requirements and the logistics of receiving, storing, preparing, and organizing the patients' food in facilities outside of the treatment units. These facilities had to meet all IPC standards and adhere to all protocols. Selected caterers were vetted in a transparent manner. Their human resource capacity to manage, distribute, and monitor patient diet and intake was carefully assessed. The IMS case management team facilitated training when and where indicated to equip catering staff with the knowledge and requisite skills to perform their tasks well.

Epidemiology and Surveillance

At the start of the outbreak, Liberia's surveillance and data collections systems were very weak. The IMS' intention was to increase surveillance and data collection and improve data entry and analysis, using information and communication technology, by the end of September 2014. We needed accurate data to make sound science-based decisions. Luke Bawo, director of MOHSW Division of Health Management Information System and Research (HMIS), was put in charge of the reinvigorated IMS Epidemiology and Surveillance (Epi-Surveillance) pillar.

Data from the MOHSW Surveillance Division indicated that by mid-August, only 25% of all reported EVD patients had been admitted to ETUs. This figure is probably underreported, considering that ETUs had an insufficient number of beds and many EVD patients did not make it to the two existing ETUs in Montserrado County or died in the lot surrounding the facility while waiting for a bed. Families, afraid of getting infected, found ways to get the sick out of their homes, leaving them in the lot to die, instead of keeping them at home. Most patients admitted to the ETU in the early stages of the epidemic died, making the case-fatality rate extremely high. A staffing shortage and inadequate training may have contributed to this high death rate.

In early October, during one of my many 8:00 a.m. operations meetings, Peter Graff, the head of the United Nations Mission for Ebola Emergency Response (UNMEER), came to my office, accompanied by Dr. Hans Rosling (now deceased), a Swedish physician, professor of international health, and former head of the Division of Global Health at the Karolinska Institute in Stockholm. Dr. Rosling was a global health celebrity and public speaker, whose riveting lectures made him a star of TED Talks and a prominent figure of the World Economic Forum in Davos, Switzerland. Dr. Rosling had come to Liberia on his own, without any organizational affiliation, because he preferred to remain independent in volunteering his services. He said he wanted to learn firsthand what was happening at the epicenter. At age sixty-six, he had no intention of working in an ETU but wanted to use his experience investigating epidemics in Africa to help with data collection, data reporting, data analysis, and presentation.

In our private discussions and in technical IMS meetings, Dr. Rosling voiced his opinions without hesitation—often speaking the truth, much to the dismay of his fellow international colleagues. One such truth he firmly believed was that, if given the knowledge and proper skill sets locally, we ourselves could bring the Ebola outbreak to a halt. In essence, we didn't need all of the fanfare that so-called international experts brought into the response, considering that most of them didn't know much about Ebola and had no "Ebola experience" to begin with. Bingo! We Liberians—physicians and members of the IMS technical teams—agreed with him 100%.

Luke Bawo had been struggling to collect data and produce daily epidemiological situation reports (sitreps) to present to IMS technical meetings every morning. They needed technical assistance, and Dr. Rosling was right there—ready, willing, and able to assist them, volunteering to do whatever was needed. On October 20, he joined Bawo's team—at first, volunteering to proofread the epidemiological reports and reorganize data reporting methods for counties that had reported zero cases.

Recognizing the extent of Dr. Rosling's expertise with data, Bawo agreed to work with him to build the capacity of his team in data collection, organization, and production of the daily sitreps. His independence as a volunteer allowed him to become fully immersed with the team, preferring to be "working for Luke as part of his team," as he would often introduce himself. In his efforts to make sense of the difficulties encountered in reporting, he spoke directly with surveillance officers in all fifteen counties. What he found was alarming: the key reason for zero reported cases in distant counties was a lack of money and tools. Daily reports were being submitted by phone, either by directly calling or by using cellular phone Internet data. The government did not provide surveillance officers with cellular phones designated specifically for reporting, nor any other means of phone access. When the surveillance officers did submit reports, they used their personal cellular phones and money to buy scratch cards to supply airtime and Internet data. However, surveillance officers responsible for calling in or submitting epidemiological data via the Internet often had no money to purchase scratch cards and refused to use their personal phones to call in reports.

To solve the problem, Dr. Rosling personally supplied the funds to make scratch cards available to surveillance officers. By closing this resource gap, surveillance officers were now motivated to do their jobs: active case finding, extensive contact tracing, and isolation of symptomatic and suspected cases. They had a daunting task in every aspect, moving from village to village, town to town, in remote locations far away from the main road. The distances were usually long—eight or ten miles, more in some cases, and only accessible by foot or motorbike. Many contacts tried to run away or hide due to the fear and stigma associated with Ebola virus infection. Surveillance officers had to track down those who sought care from traditional healers, often in thick forests. They had a hard time convincing people that they could not heal themselves and needed to be removed from the villages and isolated for supportive care and treatment.

Dr. Rosling demonstrated for us, in a flowchart, how information about patients and their contacts was disseminated through a reporting system. Data could be lost at several steps; some people died on the way to the hospital, while others gave different names, ages, or addresses. He was looking at how many of the newly discovered Ebola patients were already on one of the contact lists.

Dr. Rosling said to me in a meeting that he believed that Africa and its people were unfairly and persistently characterized by Westerners "as a continent of incompetence, superstition, and rampant corruption." He felt this projection needed to change. And, with his simple

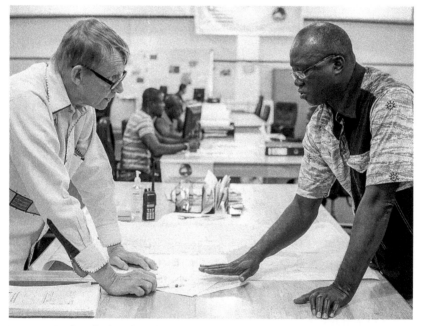

Dr. Hans Rosling (*left*) with Luke Bawo (*right*) in his office at Liberia's Ministry of Health in Monrovia. Photo by Daniel Van Moll / LAIF; https://www.sciencemag.org/news/2014/12/star-statistician-hans-rosling-takes-ebola

humanitarian act, he helped the national Ebola epi-surveillance team make sense of a major impediment in Liberia's response to the largest recorded Ebola outbreak in its history.

Community Engagement and Social Mobilization

Understanding African cultural nuances and traditional practices was critical during the Ebola epidemic. Native laws and customs are sacred and often perceived as traditional rites of passage throughout the various stages of an individual's life. For Liberians born in rural villages and towns, life was based on community or ethnic laws and customs, and elders were revered. Whatever they handed down as tradition often was accepted without question. It mattered not what others outside of the community or ethnic group thought.

When Ebola struck, no one knew what it was. The information being disseminated was confusing, especially because people were being told that the rituals that were an integral part of their lives were bad for them; if they dared continue to practice these rituals, they would get sick and die miserably, alone, without their beloved families by their side. This led to many rumors about Ebola. Some believed it was the government's fault. Some believed corrupt government officials created this myth to get money from the Europeans, Americans, and international NGOs. Some even believed that the president and her cronies were selling off the country to foreigners and brought Ebola in to kill poor people to make it easier to take their land. In other circles, Ebola was attributed to witchcraft.

Amid the confusion was widespread resistance and wholesale distrust. People became suspicious of everything the government recommended. With suspicion came rejection, putting the government in a bind. These sentiments were loudly expressed in Monrovia, in the villages, and on the farms throughout the length and breadth of Liberia, making public health interventions suspect and difficult to implement. People suspected of having EVD sought refuge and healing in churches, spiritual healing temples, and prayer houses, where pastors claimed they would be healed by the laying on of hands. This reinforced that public health messages had to be clear and simple, taking into consideration the cultural nuances—native laws and customs—of the targeted community or ethnic group.

The degree of literacy of these groups of people played a key role in the kind of messages crafted. "Many Liberians have either no formal education or only some elementary education. Forty-one percent of females and 30% of males age 6 and older have never had any formal education. Twenty-nine percent of females and 27% of males have not completed elementary schooling. Three percent of females and males have completed elementary school. Only 5% of women and 8% of men have completed senior high school. Women have completed a median of 1 year of school, while men have completed a median of 3.5 years."[11] Most of the population in villages and towns do not read or write. Pictures and graphic designs had to be considered in crafting all public health messages to more broadly target the entire population, with attention paid to the level of literacy where specific messages would be disseminated.

The government needed someone who understood the sensitivity of promoting public health messages that encouraged people to abandon traditions and practices they held dear. Reverend John Sumo, the director of risk communications and social mobilization at MOHSW, was the right man for the job. His expertise in risk communications was unparalleled in Liberia. He understood the sensitivity and risks of promoting public health messages that interfered with the community's way of living in traditional or rural settings. Sumo was appointed pillar lead for Social Mobilization and Community Engagement in Liberia's IMS in August 2014, at a time when social mobilization activities lagged far behind other aspects of the response. Medical response activities were taking shape and quarantine of several communities was underway, which made people question the government's motives more each day.

Once communication and mobilization activities became central to the response, a number of foreign and local organizations got involved, each with their own methods. Guinea, Liberia, and Sierra Leone saw an onslaught of various approaches to communication and social mobilization, which relied either on mass media or on top-down dissemination of information via social mobilizers, as opposed to ongoing grassroots-level discussions that actively solicited community perspectives and encouraged their involvement. The community had to be educated and made aware of the facts of EVD and what was fiction. This was the first time that mass community mobilization strategies were utilized in a rapidly evolving public health emergency.

To mobilize communities in the fight against Ebola, we trained approximately 10,000 volunteers, traditional leaders, chiefs, women, and youth groups.[12] We developed and distributed a key message guide for a campaign called "Ebola Must Go, It's Everybody's Business."[12,13]

Utilizing an approach to "reach every district" (RED), we trained leaders in 83% of health districts in fourteen counties in just thirty days.[12] We used the Liberian Broadcasting System (ELBC radio) and other radio stations across the country to give daily updates on EVD in local vernacular. The Knowledge, Attitudes, and Practices (KAP) survey model was employed in the field to collect close to real-time data on social behaviors and community awareness of EVD. We used the community household approach (CHA), which emphasizes that health workers and community volunteers adhere to high IPC standards to ensure their safety and that of the cases they manage. In this regard, standard operating procedures (SOPs) were drafted for all case management options, finalized September 16, and then disseminated to appropriate facilities. At the same time, home-based hygiene kits were distributed to communities nationwide.

Despite all of our efforts, community engagement remained a challenge. Our messages were not easily accepted. Community members disregarded public health messages that discouraged them from engaging in traditional practices. They remained complacent, choosing instead to believe that Ebola was nonexistent or would be short-lived. Contacts of those confirmed or suspected of having EVD were stigmatized. Even more so were those who survived the dreaded disease.

Getting the religious community to actively participate in social mobilization and community engagement could not be overemphasized. We learned by doing, incorporating adaptive interventions and innovative implementation strategies, and by reaching out to bishops, imams, and pastors to help us promulgate the messages. This was necessary, when one considers that of all Liberians in the population at the time, 84% of all women and 83% of all men were Christians; Muslim men and women constituted 14%, and 1% practiced no religion at all.[11]

Separate Ebola prevention and control guidebooks were developed for Muslin and Christian religious leaders.[14] Messages were tailored to each. We included quotes and verses from both the Holy Quran and the Holy Bible. For example, for Muslins we said, "Allah says: O you who have believed, protect yourselves and your families" (C66:6). Churches and mosques operated as communication hubs; therefore, they could provide spiritual support during the Ebola epidemic and other public health emergencies, such as COVID-19 today. They also advocated for the needs of vulnerable populations. In addition, Christian and Islamic leaders have far-reaching contacts within congregations and local communities, thereby building relationships of trust with one another. Pastors, imams, and other influential leaders in both churches and mosques served as a critical mechanism for communicating health messages about Ebola to their congregations and communities at large. Again, the same applies for COVID-19 today. In the Quran, Allah says, "O you who believe, obey Allah, and obey the messenger and those in authority among you" (C4:59). This quote helped us reinforce to the Liberian Muslims the need to respect health messages coming from the government and health authorities.

In reaching our Christian population, verses from the Bible that support infectious disease outbreak response were shared. Deuteronomy 28:61 says, "Also, every sickness, and every plague, which *is* not written in the book of this law, them will the LORD bring upon thee, until thou be destroyed." Matthew 24:7 says, "For nation shall rise against nation, and kingdom against kingdom: and there shall be famines, and pestilences, and earthquakes, in various places."

Regarding signs and symptoms, we referenced Leviticus 13:1–2: "And the Lord said unto Moses and Aaron,"[15] and "When a man shall have in the skin of his flesh a rising, a scab, or bright spot, and it be in the skin of his flesh *like* the plague of leprosy; then he shall be brought unto Aaron the priest, or unto one of his sons the priests."[16]

Field reports on social mobilization activities from counties to the IMS were slow and often incomplete. However, some reports indicated that collective community denial and aggressive resistance persisted; survivors were being intimidated and ostracized when they returned from treatment units. Therefore, it became unsafe for Ebola survivors to go home. We had to find alternative accommodations for them. We had to handle issues that threatened their existence. We needed to augment our efforts in directly engaging communities in response activities as a means of giving them some semblance of ownership in the mobilization process. By doing so, we believed we could better educate them, gain their trust, and encourage them to abandon some—if not most—of the practices that were detrimental to their health. Only then would we be able to contain the epidemic and keep infection and death rates at a minimum.

We did not undertake any impact evaluations on community mobilization in Ebola response to determine how impactful our messages were. What we had were shared experiences or lessons learned from some implementing agencies and researchers. Later in the response, there were many innovations in community mobilization that used technology, anthropological insights, and community-based research. However, there was no interagency coordination or integrations of approaches among implementing partners. Consequently, data collection and data analysis were not forthcoming to make the necessary adjustments in response activities.

There were several partner organizations:

- Mercy Corps implemented a community mobilization program called the Ebola Community Action Platform (ECAP) from December 2014 through June 2015. The program was funded by the USAID Office of Foreign Disaster Assistance (OFDA). Mercy

Corps provided sub-grants to seventy-seven partner organizations—seventy-three of which were Liberian community-based organizations. Over 800 members from partner organizations were trained in a Listen, Learn, Act methodology that emphasized listening to community concerns about Ebola, facilitated locally driven learning about the diseases and practices, and supported the development of community action plans based on what had been learned.[12] Communities then worked with their local leaders to implement these plans, such as installing handwashing stations at homes or creating a local task force to support prevention activities. Mercy Corps's subgrantee partners used this Listen, Learn, Act methodology to train more than 15,000 local community communicators, who then mobilized the members of their own villages. This allowed partner organizations the flexibility to decide the kinds of mobilization activities they would use and how they selected community educators. Using this method, Mercy Corps reported that they reached 2.4 million people, approximately 56% of the total population of Liberia.[12]

As part of the mobilization campaign, Mercy Corps implemented a technology-based monitoring and learning platform and a rapid social science research team. Partners conducted monthly random sample surveys on knowledge, attitudes, and practices in villages using smartphones donated by the Paul G. Allen Family Foundation. This allowed the program team to track the evolving attitudes of a sample of over 7,500 people reached by community mobilization.[12] A. Wa-Nyebo Neufville, an Ebola Community Action Platform (ECAP) communicator in Maryland County, said,

> One of the major challenges we were facing was about the ETU. . . . They saw it as a government attempt to bring Ebola in Maryland. It was hard to convince them. We taught them about the ETU. . . . We even encouraged some of them to go around the ETU and see what happens there and ask questions. We didn't take one day or one moment

to pause. . . . Now, I can say about 80% of the people see the ETU as important. You see, we all agree and are willing to kick Ebola out of Liberia . . . and when I see people changing their behaviors like this, it gives me more strength to continue and want to do more.[12]

The largest observed changes in attitudes over time were in acceptance of health workers who had been deployed in ETUs (from 15% to 68%) and acceptance of Ebola survivors (from 19% to 75%). The survey data indicated that by the end of the mobilization program, communities' acceptance of burial teams and messages not to touch was nearly universal.[12]

- Population Services International (PSI) provided technical expertise and training in community mobilization and communications methods. PSI also disseminated Ebola response messages among youth—"Ebola Must Go: It's Everybody's Business"—through peer-to-peer engagement, by using social marketing strategies, adapted from the "Hang Up, Keep Up" mosquito net campaign (designed to encouraged people to sleep under mosquito nets) and from their HIV campaign, promoting awareness around condom use.

- The International Research & Exchanges Board (IREX) is an international, nonprofit organization that specializes in global education and development. IREX works with partners in more than 100 countries.[17] It worked with community radio stations to complement the face-to-face mobilization with mass media messaging. The program focused on working with trusted community leaders and organizations to bridge the information gaps and promote adaptive behaviors and norms necessary to prevent the spread of Ebola. These included washing hands, not touching sick family members, and increasing community acceptance of Ebola treatment units.

- United Nations International Children's Emergency Fund (UNICEF) has been a friend and partner to Liberia for decades and has seen us through some of our darkest days during the protracted civil war. In a cross-cutting community-based approach, UNICEF engaged communities by establishing community "animation cells," which consisted of trusted individuals and networks, including religious leaders, youth and women's groups, business leaders, and Ebola survivors. UNICEF provided support to obtain survivors' testimonies to help reduce fear and encourage people to seek early treatment. Interpersonal communication was reinforced by mass communication, including regular programs on local radio stations.

Laboratory Testing

From March through July 2014, in the early stages of the outbreak, the National Reference Laboratory (NRL) had no human or technical capacity to diagnose viral hemorrhagic diseases such as Ebola. Dr. Philip Sarh, head of NRL, would carry samples from Liberia across the border, traveling by canoe into Guinea, where the samples were later flown to Lyon, France, for confirmatory diagnosis. Sometimes it took weeks if not months to get the results back. Dr. Sarh had a single laptop computer containing the Ebola test results. He alone had access to the dataset for sharing the results.

By early July, only thirty to forty specimens per day could be tested by polymerase chain reaction (PCR). Consequently, the rapidly escalating infections were neither recorded nor reported. By late July, the Liberia Institute for Biomedical Research (LIBR) was able to conduct Ebola testing, with support from the US National Institutes of Health (NIH) and the US Army Medical Research Institute of Infectious Diseases.[18] During that time, LIBR, located in Charlesville, Margibi County, housed the National Reference Laboratory, the only laboratory in the country that was conducting EVD testing. International partners, including the US military, established a temporary laboratory network to provide Ebola test results within twenty-four hours to any location in the country. The laboratory was a full day's drive from many outlying areas, and counties had very few vehicles to safely transport patients or laboratory specimens. Specimens from the ETU in Lofa County were sent across the border to Gueckedou, Guinea, for testing in the laboratory there, which was supported by the European Union.

This arrangement was threatened in mid-August by an increase in the number of specimens requiring testing and the closure of international borders. Meanwhile, there were only three functional laboratories in Liberia, located in Lofa, Monrovia, and at LIBR. IMS's objective was to increase the number of functioning laboratories from three to ten and boost both human and technical capacity by the end of October so that specimens from counties without laboratories could more easily be transported to areas with existing laboratory capacity.

By December, we had achieved our goal of having ten functioning laboratories nationwide, where real-time reverse transcription PCR testing for Ebola genomic RNA (genotyping and gene expression analysis) was available. Throughout the outbreak, adequate staffing and rapid transport of specimens remained a challenge. We sometimes had to use helicopters to transport specimens from remote areas. Later during the outbreak, the CDC brought in mobile laboratories; placement of these mobile units was determined based on facilities with available beds.

Due to administrative differences, midway in the response Dr. Sarh was replaced by Henry Korha, a laboratory technologist, to lead the Laboratory pillar, along with a team of other trained laboratory technologists who provided technical support with specimen testing, reporting, and data dissemination, which became more efficient. This enhanced the overall response rate.

Psychosocial Support

We provided psychosocial support to over 775 families in all fifteen counties.[19] As of mid-December, 2,079 affected children (998 males and 1,081 females) received support through their families or transitional homes.[20] A feedback loop telephone system was created for families to receive feedback on family members admitted to the ETU in

Montserrado County, by providing cellular phones and scratch cards to family members to call in daily. We produced and distributed a report on gaps in service provision for survivor care and recruited and trained fifty mental health workers, sixty social workers in ten counties, and fifteen city supervisors.[20] Challenges to the psychosocial support structure required strengthening linkages between psychosocial, case management, epi/surveillance, and social mobilization to ensure an integrated, comprehensive support structure for patients, survivors, and families.[20]

Dead Body Management: Safe and Dignified Burials

Ebola virus transmission occurs from direct exposure to dead bodies, so it was important to make communities aware of this risk. To prevent EVD spread, in traditional community settings the handling of dead bodies had to be completely avoided by family members. Physical preparation and burial had to be performed only by teams of people trained to safely handle and bury Ebola-infected corpses. We knew that even during this emotional period of grief, traditional practices with burial rituals had to be halted and other provisions made to allow family members to say their goodbyes to deceased relatives. Creating opportunities for safe yet dignified burials was a way to show respect for cultures and traditions and perhaps give some comfort to those left behind in their period of mourning.[21]

With all its good intention to accommodate grieving families while safely laying their loved ones to rest, the government faced major challenges with rapidly increasing cases and fatalities. There were no cemeteries with enough landmass to bury thousands of bodies in a short period of time. Logistical support was grossly inadequate. There were very few trained staff on the two burial teams to quickly collect, remove, transport, and bury Ebola-infected cadavers; they were overworked, ill-trained, and understaffed for several months into the epidemic.

With support from the International Federation of Red Cross (IFRC) and subsequently from Global Communities, burial teams in Montserrado County were increased to nineteen by mid-September 2014. Twenty-six other teams were set up in the other fourteen counties, making a national total of 45 burial teams, each charged with collecting infected corpses and conducting safe and dignified burials.[21]

After the government decided in August 2014 to cremate the bodies of those who died of EVD, the public was enraged. Following the significant backlash, the government, with the intervention of the IMS, put an end to the practice in January 2015. The IMS identified a site for a new cemetery and proposed the end of cremation to the Presidential Ebola Advisory Council. The president visited the site and agreed to reverse the mandatory order. After heated negotiations with community leaders on the price of the land, the Disco Hill Cemetery officially opened in January 2015, with a team of grave diggers trained to work with the burial teams. The public was more accepting of this government decision and more likely to cooperate. The government subsequently closed down its crematories and opened a cemetery at Disco Hill in Margibi County, off the highway that leads to Roberts International Airport (RIA).

The Disco Hill burial ground then became the new national cemetery, initially intended for safe and dignified burials of those who died from Ebola. There were two separate designated burial areas, one for Christians and the other for Muslims. This allowed families to accompany burial teams that carried their loved ones to the cemetery. Families traveled in separate vehicles, and from a distance of six to eight feet they could watch the burial being conducted. Some chose to perform burial rites from where they stood or sat in their vehicles.

Nationally, the burial team was headed by Mark Y. Korvayan. Adequate burial teams and burial sites were established in communities in each of the fifteen counties. Fifty 4 × 4 pickup trucks were procured to collect the dead and an additional fifty Toyota 4 × 4 vehicles were added to this fleet. Consequently, burials became more systematic after Disco Hill and other cemeteries were identified and established in other parts of the country.

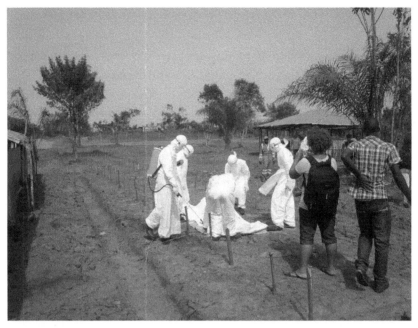

Disco Hill Cemetery. Dead Body Management Team preparing a corpse for burial.
Photo courtesy of the Ministry of Health and Social Welfare, Republic of Liberia

Logistics and Support Services

The Logistics pillar dealt with ordering, distributing, maintaining, replacing, and returning items that were not being used to the warehouse. Dorbor Jallah, the Logistics pillar lead, oversaw ETU construction, ambulance services, dead body management, cargo clearing, food distribution, and emergency call centers.[22] The logistics team provided storage at a hub at RIA (the airport), with a capacity of 145,673 cubic feet. However, the main logistics base was located at the Samuel Kanyon Doe (SKD) Sports Complex, with a capacity of 129,251 cubic feet.[22] Furthermore, forward logistics bases (FLB), with total capacity of 302,576 cubic feet, were built in the south, east, north, central, western, and southeastern regions of Liberia. Nine mobile storage units (MSUs), with total capacity of 88,286 cubic feet, were constructed and functional. These logistics resources were placed at the disposal of the logistic teams: (1) transport and fuel capacity long-haul trucks; (2) twenty-nine flatbed long-haul trucks (twenty 4×6 and nine 6×6 trucks); (3) ten local transport contracts by the World Food Programme, and (4) fifty-nine trucks with the capacity of 2,000 metric tons (MT) were used to transport Ebola goods to faraway places (the last mile). A total of forty Dutch Truck Manufacturing (DAF) last-mile trucks were assigned to serve the main logistics base (MLB) and port hub; twenty-eight DAF trucks supported the airport hub, while two DAF trucks, for each of the FLBs to support the counties, were used (for example, in the southeastern region, which was very hard to reach).[22]

The magnitude of the logistics challenge cut across major operational areas: Ebola treatment units, community care centers, laboratories, health facilities, incoming donations from various worldwide sources, multiple owners, infrastructure challenges (roads, ICT, etc.), and a lack of demand data. As part of the logistics effort, items were assembled and dispatched from the MLB and FLBs to remote hotspots. International partners, the World Food Programme in particular, helped to facilitate the movement of humanitarian passengers and cargo throughout Liberia, utilizing assets such as helicopters and fixed-wing airplanes. A key part of the partners' support included transporting blood samples by air and an unprecedented supply of medical equipment (gloves, face masks, plastic aprons). In addition to realizing that the crisis needed one response with a unitary command structure and locals in charge, we saw the necessity for a single supply chain leadership, with pooled resources.

Finance and Administration

IMS's Finance and Administration pillar provided services to initiate, operate, and sustain the emergency operations center. I appointed Miatta Gbanya as a principal deputy incident manager for administration and finance. As she said, "the health workforce is the core of any epidemic response."[23]

Health Care Workers

Hazard pay was initiated in September 2014 after the landmark agreement on the rates per category was reached through negotiations led by the Ministry of Finance and Development Planning, the Ministry of Health, the Liberia Medical and Dental Council Boards of Directors, and leadership of various health care workers' associations. Although an agreement was signed, there was still a lot of dissatisfaction among health workers regarding pay rates and status of employment. The issue was further analyzed and a briefing paper presented to the Presidential Advisory Council on Ebola (PACE), which emphasized that the problem could not possibly be resolved during the EVD epidemic as it was linked to ongoing unresolved human resource issues.[24] After the PACE meeting on November 3, the deputy minister for administration and the chief medical officer, together with the IMS team, sent a communication to partners and county health officers based on the decision reached.

An additional financial grant from the World Bank, referred to as Emergency Ebola Response Project–Additional Financing (EERP–AF) and valued at US$115 million, was signed in October 2014 and ended in September 2015 with possibility of extension, based on discussions between the government of Liberia (Ministry of Health [MOH] and Ministry of Finance and Development Planning [MOFDP], managed through the Public Financial Management Unit [PFMU] at MOFDP) and the World Bank.[25] This grant had a minimum amount for local hazard pay and a substantial amount for recruitment and payment of foreign medical teams and international responders managed by UNOPS and WHO. The amount for local hazard pay fell under component 2 of the EERP–AF EVD Care (Community Care Center) in the amount of US$2,865,780. The support targeted health care workers and response personnel in Ebola treatment units. UNDP also supported operations related to hazard payments for Ebola responders and routine health care workers, covering the period from October 2014 to March 2015.

The payment process was complicated, and there were several issues that were later identified as lessons to be learned:

- New lists had to be generated for response teams and the county health teams.
- Duplications of names, account numbers, and wrong account numbers were problematic.
- The payment process required a bank account for easy transfer of payment, otherwise cutting checks or paying with cash (in some instances) would delay the process further. A considerable number of people did not have active bank accounts or had never owned one. They were encouraged to open bank accounts, and many of them did.
- Contracts were issued or reissued—getting all contracts signed was a requirement for payment.
- Payment lists for county health teams and response teams had to be checked and verified to prevent corruption.
- Deployment of pay teams to counties and recording time of work for payment had to be carefully monitored.
- Death benefits requirements had to be agreed upon and clarified for deceased workers and their families.
- An existing workforce payment issue—the classification as civil servant versus non-civil servant versus contractor, which determined pay rate—was challenged.[23]

The HR team had limited staffing capacity and was overwhelmed with backlogs of delayed payments, poor and delayed communication with the teams on hazard pay, and no payment made to workers of private health facilities. All of these problems grew more complicated each day as further delays in hazard payment were distressing to all concerned. As we implemented the exit plan when the response officially ended, these issues had to be resolved if we were to have a smooth transition. The difficulties surrounding hazard pay, HR, and regular payroll were handled by Miatta Gbanya, my deputy for finance. Like many other response workers, she was magnanimous.

Airport, Seaport, and Land Borders

The Ebola epidemic had begun with the disease crossing borders be-tween Guinea, Liberia, and Sierra Leone. In July 2014, it spread to Ni-geria. The CDC advised the Liberian government to set up entry and exit screening at Roberts International Airport (RIA) / Robertsfield in Margibi, County, to enhance safety and continuity of air traffic into and out of Liberia. Enhanced screening procedures and protocols were im-plemented at Robertsfield. All incoming and outgoing passengers had temperature screenings. On the advice of the CDC, Liberian epidemi-ologists and surveillance officers considered creating a travel restriction list using MOHSW's EVD database or other available information; at the time, implementing intensive screening procedures was difficult because the airport facilities were not equipped and the staffing capa-bilities were limited. The IMS team collaborated with airline companies to augment health security procedures, training ground and air staff to evaluate and possibly isolate passengers who were denied boarding for suspicious health concerns. At the seaports, border control proce-dures were further enhanced. In early August, as the epidemic wors-ened, the government imposed isolation of Lofa County. The borders with Sierra Leone and Guinea were closed. Certain communities in Lofa and Bomi Counties voluntarily isolated themselves.

To implement stricter air, sea, and land border controls and screen-ing, the government provided material and logistics, trained existing personnel, and aggressively recruited staff to increase capacity at the ports of entry. The government also negotiated with air carriers to pro-vide air transport in and out of Liberia. Almost all major and regional airlines ceased flying to Liberia for fear of infecting their staff or trans-porting infected persons and spreading Ebola globally. Brussels Airlines was the only international carrier that continued flying to Liberia throughout and after the Ebola response. For this, President Sirleaf honored Brussels Airlines with Liberia's Order of the Star of Africa, with the Grade of Commander.[26]

The International Response

Agencies within the international community that were regarded as having all the expertise and technical know-how often proved disappointing. Many of their representatives had never dealt with an Ebola outbreak—and definitely not one of this magnitude or in an urban metropolis. All previous Ebola outbreaks had been on a much smaller scale, in remote and rural villages along the Ebola River in the Democratic Republic of the Congo. During discussions in incident management system meetings, we at the MOHSW were appalled to learn that members of the WHO, CDC, MSF teams, and others had never handled an Ebola situation—ever. This experience was new to most of those who had come, and this lack of expertise or direct experience with Ebola or an Ebola response created a lot of anxiety in those of us who were charged with managing our country's response. All the blame for the poor response had been placed on the WHO, which had provided overall technical advice on the direction the response would take, and the Liberian government, whose leadership for the outbreak was uncoordinated and had been declared inept. But these attacks came from the so-called experts, who said they came to help despite admittedly not knowing much about handling Ebola themselves. We were all in the same boat, Liberians and internationals alike. The situation was new to everyone.

The international community had been slow to respond to our plight. Biosecurity and global health were their paramount concerns only after foreigners working in Liberia became infected. Evacuations were arranged to the United States and Spain. Then suddenly there was a heightened interest in the trans-Atlantic spread of Ebola. Biosecurity is defined as "the prevention of disease-causing agents entering or leaving any place where they can pose a risk to farm animals, other animals, humans, or the safety and quality of a food product."[1] Good biosecurity should be practiced at all times, not just during a disease outbreak.[1] It was then that the concepts of the Global Health Security Agenda (GHSA) and biosecurity were introduced to Liberia. GHSA emphasizes the importance of a whole-of-government and multisectoral effort to build national capacity to prepare for biological catastrophes, which includes human and animal health, agriculture, security, defense, and law enforcement.[2] The United States has been a longstanding global health security leader. In 2014, the United States helped launch the GHSA to strengthen the world's ability to prevent, detect, and respond to infectious disease threats.[2] Now, more than seventy countries as well as international organizations, nongovernmental organizations, and private sector entities are united in a common goal of measurably strengthening global health security—with the target of strengthening country capacities by 2024 for 100 countries in at least three broad areas:[2] prevent avoidable epidemics, including naturally occurring outbreaks and intentional or accidental releases; detect threats early, including detecting, characterizing, and transparently reporting emerging biological threats at the earliest possible moment; and respond rapidly and effectively to biological threats of international concern.[3,4]

Subsequently, in Liberia, a national version of the GHSA roadmap was developed in 2015:[5]

- A structure for multisectorial collaboration and coordination was established using the One Health approach, which recognizes the link between the health of humans, animals, and the environment.

- Approximately 14,000 health care workers were trained in infection prevention and control practices.
- IDSR (Integrated Disease Surveillance and Response) reporting was implemented across the fifteen counties and ninety-two districts.
- Community event-based surveillance (CEBS) was established: community health workers (CHWs) identify disease outbreaks, alert and report to the surveillance system by using visual aids (pictures, drawings, etc.) because most CHWs are barely educated or not educated at all.
- The Community Health Assistance Program (CHAP) was launched, which recruits, trains, and provides support for CHWs that perform functions such as integrated management of childhood illnesses (malaria, acute respiratory infections, diarrhea, and immunizations) at the community level.
- A weekly epidemiological bulletin was introduced.
- National and county-specific Epidemic Preparedness and Response plans were developed.[5]

By October, more than 4,500 people across West Africa had died of the dreaded disease, including 2,200 in Liberia, making Liberia the epicenter of the epidemic. In Guinea, Liberia, and Sierra Leone, approximately 9,000 people were confirmed positive for Ebola and it was estimated that 70% of the infected would perish. However, by 2016, when the WHO officially declared the epidemic had "ended in the human population," fatality rates in the West African epidemic had reached only 50%.[6,7,8]

On October 19, 2014, in an open letter to the world, President Sirleaf wrote, "This is a fight in which the whole world has a stake. This disease respects no borders. . . . Across West Africa, a generation of young people risk being lost to economic catastrophe. . . . This fight requires a commitment from every nation that has the capacity to help."[9]

What Liberia needed most was strong leadership, clearly defined strategies, and protocols to avert transmission. Communities across the country needed to be engaged in order to take ownership of controlling the outbreak. And resources were needed—human and material—which the international community brought later.

World Health Organization

The WHO was the established lead technical partner in health to the government of Liberia, long before the outbreak. As such, the agency retained this role on the Incident Management Team. The WHO team was always in the room, with a seat at the table, cross-cutting all thematic pillars and providing overall technical support and training for health workers; mobile laboratories and lab supplies; constructing Ebola treatment units; and supporting contact tracing, case management, and dead body management teams. Personnel changes of top-level officials were made at its Country Office within a short span of time. The WHO team was first headed by Dr. Nestor Ndayimirije, then by Peter Graff, and finally by Dr. Alex Gasasira, who each played important roles at every stage in the outbreak response. Dr. Gasasira had previously worked in Liberia as a WHO consultant for the Expanded Programme on Immunization (EPI), and he understood the country's health system and its social and economic context pre-Ebola. Consequently, he was magnanimous, bringing vigor and efficiency to the response overall. The changes appeared unplanned and very abrupt. We believed that deficiencies or inconsistencies in the initial WHO response, which handicapped the overall national response, dictated these changes.

On August 28, Bruce Aylward, the WHO assistant director-general, projected that there could be 20,000 cases of Ebola virus in West Africa and that the numbers could double or quadruple in some areas before the outbreak ended.[10] At that time, there were already 3,000 confirmed cases in the region. Of this number, 1,552 people had died in the three most affected countries (Guinea, Liberia, and Sierra Leone) and Nigeria.[11]

Following the spread of Ebola from Liberia to Nigeria in July, regional airlines canceled flights to and from our country. This travel ban hindered response efforts as we could not travel out and no one could travel into Liberia. Therefore, supplies could not easily be brought in. People who wanted to help were afraid to come to Liberia. Relief organizations did not want to risk exposing their staff to the deadly disease. There were too many potential liabilities. We faced a serious predicament. At this point, WHO made an appeal to all airlines that provided flights across West Africa, encouraging them to resume regional service and lift the travel ban. If they did not, the threat of Ebola would intensify and compromise response efforts. WHO's appeal was supported by African ministers of health attending a meeting convened by the Economic Community of West African States (ECOWAS) in Accra, Ghana. They called on member states to reopen their borders and airlines to resume regional flights.[10]

WHO also formulated a nine-month strategy for the response, projected at costing US$489 million (£295m). This strategy estimated that 12,000 West Africans and 750 foreign nationals were needed to constitute the workforce necessary for its implementation.[10] The goal, then, was to appeal to member states of the WHO to pledge financial support in the shortest time possible so that response efforts could be accelerated.

In September, WHO began renovating a 150-bed treatment center at Island Clinic on Bushrod Island. This was a turning point in the outbreak response, giving us the capacity to accommodate more Ebola patients. Teams of 100 construction workers labored around the clock in shifts, racing to complete the center. On September 21, WHO formally handed over the Island Clinic to the MOHSW. Within twenty-four hours after opening, the clinic was overflowing with patients, further demonstrating the desperate need for more treatment beds. The day before the facility was opened, a few of my colleagues and I spent the entire day and night at Island Clinic setting up mattresses and making beds.

WHO also supported the construction of two additional Ebola treatment centers, augmenting Monrovia's treatment capacity by another

400 beds. In Lofa, staff from the WHO Country Office, headed by Dr. Peter Clement, an epidemiologist (now country representative of the WHO Liberia Country Office), moved from village to village, challenging chiefs and religious leaders to take charge of their response. Several community task forces were formed to create house-to-house awareness, report suspected cases, call health teams for support, and conduct contact tracing.

African Union

On August 19, the Peace and Security Council (PSC) of the African Union (AU) held its 450th meeting, in Addis Ababa, Ethiopia, at which time it authorized the immediate deployment of an AU humanitarian mission for the effective control of Ebola and the normalization of health services in Guinea, Liberia, and Sierra Leone. The resolutions of the meeting included the following:

1. Immediate establishment of the African Union Support to Ebola in West Africa (ASEOWA), aimed at bringing out the African solidarity to respond to their own member states under the EVD pressure.
2. Mobilizing the civil, military, medical, and non-medical Ebola response operation.
3. Informing the member states of the decision to establish a Center for Disease Control (CDC) for Africa to enhance the medical capability and research on the challenges Africa is facing with diseases, to start assessing and discussing the post Ebola socio-economic recovery phase for the affected countries.
4. Promote bilateral and multilateral relationships between African member states in planning for the recovery process after Ebola.[12]

By September 12, affected countries began receiving volunteer health workers from other African countries. In total, Liberia received 265 ASEOWA health workers from Burundi, Ethiopia, the Democratic Republic of the Congo (DRC), Kenya, Nigeria, Rwanda, and Uganda. President

Sirleaf stated, "To the governments and people of these countries, Liberia would eternally be grateful." The ASEOWA team worked closely with local personnel to investigate and detect Ebola cases, trace and follow-up contacts, treat patients infected with Ebola, educate the community, provide routine health services, and train local health personnel.[12] They supported efforts to restore essential health services. The first cohort of volunteers to affected countries consisted of eighteen professionals from Nigeria, the DRC, Ethiopia, Uganda, and Rwanda.

Dr. Jean-Jacques Muyembe, the Congolese epidemiologist who first discovered Ebola in 1976, was among the first ASEOWA team members from the DRC. Dr. Muyembe was called to "an outbreak of a mysterious disease in central Congo" along the Ebola River in 1976, in Zaire, which had only recently attained independence from Belgium.[13] He was the first to collect viral samples from infected persons, which were later sent to Belgium for analysis.[14] The Belgians, including the now renowned Dr. Peter Piot, took credit as discoverers of the virus and named it Ebola, after the river region where it originated. In typical Western colonialist fashion, Dr. Muyembe was never acknowledged as the original discoverer of the Ebola virus. Zaire subsequently became the DRC in May 1997.[15] Liberia was blessed with Dr. Muyembe's presence and expertise, along with his team of five other Congolese health professionals, consisting of a medic, two nurses, a laboratory specialist, and an epidemiologist, who graciously shared their experiences with us and assisted us in formulating our response strategies and interventions. This was a turning point that tremendously impacted the success of our Ebola response.

Due to the disastrous effects of the Ebola crisis, in discussions with a small IMS team in Monrovia, President Sirleaf proposed that an Africa Centres for Disease Control and Prevention (ACDC) be established. She championed the cause alongside her newly appointed minister of health, Dr. Bernice Dahn, who succeeded Dr. Walter Gwenigale after he retired during the outbreak. They also advocated for the establishment of the National Public Health Institute of Liberia (NPHIL). Their advocacy prompted African health ministers (West African ministers

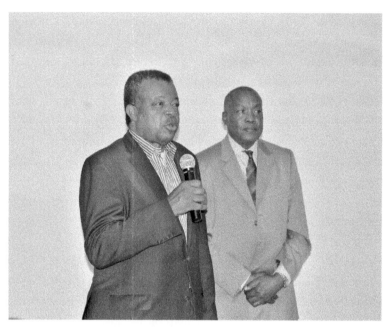

Dr. Jean-Jacques Muyembe (heading DRC delegation; *left*) and Dr. Nestor Ndayimirije (WHO country representative; *right*) at the Ebola strategy meeting in Monrovia in August 2014

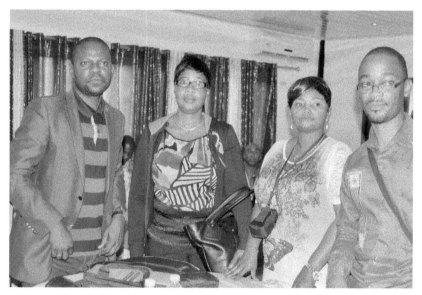

DRC team of medical professionals that accompanied Dr. Jean-Jacques Muyembe to Liberia of health, in particular) to agree on establishing the ACDC and regional collaborating centers, as well as national public health institutes across the continent. I engaged Minister Dahn and President Sirleaf to advocate with their colleagues for the headquarters to be based in Guinea, Liberia, or Sierra Leone—countries that bore the brunt of the social and economic devastation of Ebola. It made sense to me that those who suffered the most should receive the support to rebuild their weak health systems. Already, Nigeria was host to the ECOWAS headquarters and Ethiopia was host to the AU headquarters, so it was only natural to give one of the devastated countries the opportunity to host the ACDC or the regional CDC. But ultimately, Nigeria and Ethiopia were chosen as the West African regional hub and headquarters, respectively.

United States Government

The US ambassador to Liberia, Deborah Malac, declared Liberia a humanitarian disaster on August 4, prompting the deployment of a USAID Disaster Assistance Response Team (DART) to Monrovia to assess the situation.[16,17] Ambassador Malac had toured Monrovia with President Sirleaf and me to assess the burden of the Ebola virus disease. US CDC director Tom Frieden also made two visits, in August and September. Ambassador Malac attended several IMS meetings, as well as the Presidential Advisory Council on Ebola (PACE) meetings, to get a better sense of what the overall international response required. Frieden and Malac reached out to the US Congress and officials in the National Security Council, advocating for assistance to Liberia. Following a personal appeal by President Sirleaf, US President Barack Obama deployed the US military to Liberia to provide logistical support. Seeing American troops in Monrovia gave Liberians a psychological boost. This initiative was the result of collective efforts by Presidents Alpha Condé (Guinea), Ernest Bai Koroma (Sierra Leone), and Ellen Johnson Sirleaf (Liberia), pleading to the world to rescue their respective countries and the Mano River basin from the brunt of infection, potential annihilation, and economic devastation.

Ambassador Malac wanted to ensure that the Liberian government provided a suitable space, either a football stadium, very large buildings, or land space, to construct Ebola treatment units. Through her influence, we identified the old Defense Ministry site in Congo Town, the Samuel Kanyon Doe (SKD) Sports Complex in Paynesville, Island Clinic on Bushrod Island, Unity Conference Center in Virginia (on the outskirts of Monrovia), and the site that became the Monrovia Medical Center, as potential ETU sites.

When aid was forthcoming, the ambassador assured Liberians that the American military assistance was not a prelude to a coup d'état, as many citizens had expressed. Malac noted that the coordinated efforts were intended to curb the epidemic, not initiate regime change. I was thrilled that she attended IMS meetings and broadened our perspective. There were those who contributed immensely to my work as incident manager and made it easy for me. Ambassador Malac was one such person. She played a significant role in the fight against Ebola in Liberia, where her journey as US ambassador had begun in 2012. In September 2015, at the height of the epidemic, Malac left Liberia to become the US ambassador to Uganda, leaving the USAID to coordinate the US government Ebola response in Liberia.

During the epidemic, Dr. Kevin De Cock was also the US CDC's country director in Kenya. He was on rotation in and out of Liberia, along with other CDC team members. On July 16, the first members of a CDC team arrived in Monrovia to assess the extent of our preparedness to effectively manage an outbreak. Within a month, the team visited six counties with reported Ebola virus disease cases, as well as four counties with no reported cases. Working with county health teams, they visited and assessed large health facilities and investigated a number of clusters of EVD. Dr. De Cock helped me understand my role as incident manager and chairman of the IMS. Through his counsel and mentorship, I was able to handle my fears and concerns about the responsibility I had assumed, and it became easier for me to lead the response as the incident manager. His presence made a significant difference at this pivotal moment in my life. For that, I am eternally grateful.

On September 16, President Obama spoke at the CDC, where he made a surprise announcement that a 3,000-member US military force was being deployed to West Africa. Operation United Assistance (OUA) was led by Major General Darryl Williams, commander of the United States Army Africa, who had arrived in Liberia twenty-four hours before the announcement.[17] Major General Williams and thirteen other officers were on an initial fact-finding mission. President Sirleaf convened a meeting in her office at the Executive Mansion in Monrovia, to which she invited the IMS team, Ambassador Malac, and Major General Williams. This was our introductory meeting with the general. He informed us that his mission was to support the civilian government. This was welcome news because many in the country speculated that American troops had come to Liberia to assassinate President Sirleaf to force a regime change in the midst of a crisis.

Critical elements in the strategy to contain the Ebola outbreak included setting up ETUs and the Monrovia Medical Unit, and isolating EVD patients by removing confirmed, suspected, and probable cases from the general population and providing relevant supportive treatment. Liberia needed functioning ETUs as quickly as possible; the Disaster Assistance Response Team (DART) presented the task to the US Department of Defense (DOD) on September 25, which directed the DOD to build up to seventeen ETUs.[17] A number of obstacles impacted the effort, including determining an appropriate design, site selection, dealing with the rainy season, infrastructure (i.e., the physical building, including building materials, water and sewage systems, and electrical), adjusting the construction requirements as the disease pattern changed, and staffing health care workers. Establishing effective coordination among the wide variety of stakeholders was essential in solving these challenges.

Building an ETU is not as simple as erecting a tent. If it isn't done correctly, it can be lethal for the patients and the health care workers. And there was no standard ETU design to start the effort. US Army Captain Andrew Hill, one of three DOD planners embedded into DART, designed what would eventually become the ETU standard for OUA.

The process to design and build ETUs demonstrated the strong cooperation between WHO, MSF, USAID/DART, MOHSW, and DOD. WHO shared its ETU requirements and MSF invited US military engineers to visit their ETUs and explained their setup and offered their expertise. I was involved in the design modification where necessary, finding potential sites for ETUs and working with the US government officials. Finally, the US Army Corps of Engineers (USACE) and USAID/DART representatives developed ETU building plans specifically designed to be functional and feasible in the West African environment. The design met the MOHSW clinical requirements, and the elasticity of the design allowed ETUs to be adapted to various locales and conditions.

Site selection was a challenge. The original MOHSW plan was to put an ETU in each county, but actual site selection was influenced by the need for community buy-in, local infrastructure, access to water, the type of terrain, and available construction skills. Potential sites ranged from private industrial locations to mid-jungle clearings. The need for early on-site reconnaissance and input from all ETU stakeholders was an important lesson. Some sites were too small for the standard design and were modified to increase the ETU's distance between confirmed and unconfirmed cases. In addition, water wells remained a limiting factor throughout the operation, even though DOD hired every available well drilling company.[18,19]

As the lead coordinator for the US government's international disaster response, USAID's Office of Foreign Disaster Assistance (USAID/OFDA) served as the backbone of the US EVD response, coordinating efforts among other US government entities that provided needed expertise, including the CDC, the US military, NIH, and the US Public Health Service (USPHS). USAID/OFDA contributed to the response through financial and operational support to over thirty regional and local implementing partners, technical support to national response systems, and coordination of these programs with other resources committed to the response. Through USAID, the US government deployed a field-based Disaster Assistance Response Team (DART) on August 5 and established a corresponding Response Management Team (RMT) based in Washington, DC. The DART—comprising disaster response, public health, and medical experts from USAID/OFDA and CDC—worked on coordinating the interagency response and identifying key needs stemming from the EVD outbreak, in order to amplify humanitarian response efforts and lead US government efforts to support the EVD response. While USAID/OFDA coordinated the US government's overall response, the CDC provided vital technical leadership and guidance in the areas of surveillance, epidemiology, and infection prevention and control. From August 2014 to December 2016, USAID/OFDA provided more than US$809 million across the three countries to UN agencies, NGO implementers, and contractors supporting critical interventions such as health and humanitarian coordination; case management; surveillance and epidemiology; restoration of essential health services through infection prevention and control measures; water, sanitation, and hygiene (WASH) interventions; social mobilization and communications; and logistics activities, including the procurement of personal protective equipment and relief commodities. In addition, USAID/OFDA provided support to critical training activities for health care workers focused on case management, infection prevention and control, and contact tracing.[20]

US National Institutes of Health (NIH)

One important aspect of my many responsibilities as incident manager was to oversee the collaboration and/or partnership, leading to the discovery of vaccines and therapeutics to treat Ebola. Strategically, the government of Liberia's goal was to find a permanent solution, such as vaccines and therapeutic control measures, that would be complementary and/or synergistic to the traditional public health measures, such as testing and contact tracing, presumptive treatment of Ebola in ETUs or isolation, infection prevention and control, community engagement/social mobilization, and managing the dead. The permanent solution the government sought was development of medical countermeasures. Medical countermeasures, or MCMs, are defined by the CDC as "life-saving medicines and medical supplies regulated by the U.S. Food and Drug Administration (FDA) that can be used to diagnose, prevent, protect from, or treat conditions associated with chemical, biological, radiological, or nuclear (CBRN) threats, emerging infectious diseases, or a natural disaster."[21] Consequently, the government reached out to its US counterparts through the secretary of health and human services, Department of Health and Human Services (DHHS).

This effort established a multimillion-dollar research enterprise between the Liberian and United States governments, called the Partnership for Research on Ebola Virus in Liberia, or PREVAIL. PREVAIL began its operations in October 2014 at the request of Liberia's minister of health, Dr. Walter T. Gwenigale, "to develop a partnership between the Department of Health and Human Services (DHHS) and the Government of Liberia (GoL), to conduct clinical research on promising therapeutics for Ebola and vaccines for its prevention."[22] The US secretary of DHHS, then Sylvia Burwell, responded by expressing her commitment to help "combat the Ebola epidemic" and appointed Dr. H. Clifford Lane, deputy director of the National Institute of Allergy and Infectious Diseases (NIAID), to represent the DHHS research efforts.[22] The partnership was conceived during the largest and most complex Ebola outbreak since the virus was discovered, in 1976.[23]

I appointed a team of Liberians including the first head of PREVAIL research team, Dr. Stephen B. Kennedy and Dr. Fatoma Bolay (deceased), as co-principal investigators (PI). Dr Kennedy—trained in medicine—was a researcher focused on infectious disease epidemiology, behavioral science, biomedical research (HIV pathogenesis), and tuberculosis (TB). Dr. Bolay was a research scientist who worked on river blindness and schistosomiasis, retired from the WHO, and was director of the Liberia Institute for Biomedical Research (LIBR) at the time of this appointment. Both were well suited for the job. They joined their US counterparts, headed by Dr. Lane. PREVAIL became an opportunity to foster the culture of clinical research in Liberia, because we insisted on a south-north collaborative model. We also created the IMS Research Thematic Group as a response pillar. Scientists from the United States collaborated in numerous interesting scientific research initiatives, including but not limited to protocol development, data analysis, information sharing, manuscript writing, resources mobilization, logistics and operational management, and publications. In 2018, the Partnership for Research on Ebola Vaccine in Liberia was renamed Partnership for Research, Vaccines and Infectious Diseases in Liberia. However, despite this change, the acronym PREVAIL is still being used.

However, getting PREVAIL organized from the beginning was a challenge because Liberians believed that they were being used as guinea pigs by the West. Furthermore, the initial stage of the Ebola vaccine trial was characterized by community resistance. Civil society organizations demanded answers, and the Liberian society, including politicians, government officials, and community members, all were agitated. The paradox was that these were the same people who were calling for help at the peak of the outbreak. It took intensive social mobilization, lobbying, and community engagement, explaining the risks and benefits of vaccines and clinical trials, to calm the agitated community. We had to clearly explain that the benefits of the vaccine trials far exceeded the risks.

By February 2, 2015, the first participant enrolled in PREVAIL I: a phase II/III randomized, double-blind, placebo-controlled study of the chimpanzee adenovirus 3 (ChAd3-EBO-Z) vaccine and the recombinant vesicular stomatitis virus (rVSVΔG-ZEBOV-GP) vaccine.[22] Enrollment of 1,500 participants was completed by the end of April.[22] PREVAIL was also a part of a multicenter, multinational, randomized safety and efficacy study of putative investigational therapeutics in the treatment of patients with known Ebola infection (MCM RCT in EBOV) that studied ZMapp. The study was known in Liberia as PREVAIL II.[22] As the vaccine trial continued, it became evident that those who survived Ebola might experience long-term health problems. The partnership then embarked on PREVAIL III and PREVAIL IV: a Cohort Study of Survivors of Ebola Virus Infection in Liberia, semen and other sequalae.[22]

When the outbreak receded, I continued to provide executive leadership as head of the Executive Committee of PREVAIL. PREVAIL was organized in a way that it has the governing board, which was the highest level of governance within PREVAIL, providing broad strategic direction and oversight. Thus, represented at this level was the president of Liberia and the US ambassador. The second highest level of leadership in PREVAIL was the Executive Committee (EC)—which I chaired from October 2014 through November 2019. The EC represented the varied interests of the partners to reach consensus on PREVAIL strategic objectives. In addition, the EC approved new partners and budgets, established and communicated the PREVAIL overarching strategy, oversaw performance of PREVAIL, and advocated for PREVAIL members. The EC regularly assessed progress against goals, assisted with removing barriers to progress, and held the PREVAIL steering committees accountable to achieve success. There were several steering committees (finance, science, behavior change, etc.). The PREVAIL Science and Strategic Partnership Committee (PSSPC) focused on scientific reviews, research protocols, and strategic planning. During my tenure, the EC resolved conflicts when requested to do so by a steering committee. Other layers of PREVAIL management included the Operations & Management Team and subject matter experts.

The findings from the Ebola vaccine trial, as carried out by PREVAIL, was groundbreaking in the fight against Ebola. I say this because, on October 12, 2017, two years after the end of the outbreak, an article was published in the *New England Journal of Medicine* with a concluding paragraph: "A randomized, placebo-controlled phase 2 trial of two vaccines that was rapidly initiated and completed in Liberia showed the capability of conducting rigorous research during an outbreak. By 1 month after vaccination, the vaccines had elicited immune responses that were largely maintained through 12 months."[24] There was a tremendous effort put into this research, and it was successful thanks to the funders: the National Institute of Allergy and Infectious Diseases and the Liberian Ministry of Health.

Because of the vaccine research in Liberia and Guinea, vaccination is a tool in the toolbox to respond to global Ebola control efforts. Recently, the tenth and eleventh Ebola outbreaks in DRC were not as catastrophic when compared to the West African Ebola outbreak.[25] As of January 13, 2020, there were over "3,400 confirmed Ebola cases in the DRC and over 2,200 reported Ebola deaths. Over 223,000 Congolese were vaccinated and received the vaccine for Ebola, rVSV-ZEBOVGP."[25] In addition to the vaccine, the WHO also reported the discovery of two Ebola treatments being used in the DRC as part of a clinical trial which, "when used at the right time, have been shown to save 9 out of 10 lives which are the second largest in history."[25] In fact, deployment of those lifesaving innovations enabled the Guinean Health Ministry to contain a second Ebola outbreak in 2021, when just sixteen confirmed cases were reported and twelve people died. The limited size of the flare up in Guinea is attributable to the painful lessons learned from the Ebola epidemic in West Africa.[26] By June 19, 2021, WHO declared an end to the second Ebola outbreak in Guinea; the outbreak this time lasted for only five months and claimed twelve lives, according to a press statement from the WHO.[26,27]

Médecins Sans Frontières (Belgium)

Médecins Sans Frontières Belgium (MSF-B; Doctors Without Borders, representing and supported by Belgium), came to Liberia in late March and early April, primarily to support the Ministry of Health in devising plans for a response. The MSF team previously based in Sierra Leone managing viral hemorrhagic fever, was redirected across the border with some personal protection materials and was the first to arrive in Guéckédou, Guinea, on March 18. It was not until mid-August, however, that their activities in Monrovia became clearer. They committed to three main tasks: First, set up an ETU to isolate patients infected or suspected of having EVD to reduce morbidity and mortality, and protecting all ETU personnel by providing them with PPEs. Second, engage community mobilization and health promotion by educating communities about Ebola—how it is transmitted, how infections can be prevented, and if infected, how, when, and where to go for care; MSF also intended to learn more about cultural practices and traditions that could contribute to the spread of the disease. Third, provide disinfection and protection kits to households to reduce or prevent further spread of Ebola.[28]

The MSF Ebola Treatment Unit, commonly referred to as ELWA 3, began operations on August 18 with 120 beds. By September 26, an additional 130 beds were added. At that time, there were 50 suspected cases and 200 confirmed positive patients in ELWA 3. By September 28,932 suspected Ebola cases had been admitted. Eighty-five percent or 790 tested positive and 142 were negative for Ebola virus. Those confirmed positive were transferred to an isolated area of the ETU designated solely for Ebola positive patients. Patients who became completely free of symptoms were considered recovered. However, they were kept in the ETU for another two weeks, during which time they were tested each week for Ebola virus. If they tested negative for two consecutive weeks, they were discharged as Ebola survivors. Survivors were then regularly monitored for post-recovery symptoms and disability. A total of 203 survivors were discharged home during this period.[28]

In managing ELWA3, MSF-B saw confirmed Ebola cases as well as those with symptoms that mimicked Ebola. They found that 30%–40% of these cases tested negative for Ebola. A number of these patients needed to be hospitalized for diseases unrelated to Ebola but because hospitals in Liberia were functioning at a minimum, there was no place to refer them to for more comprehensive treatment or admission.

By October 19, WHO had reported a total of 4,665 Ebola infected cases in Liberia and 2,705 deaths.[29] Forty-four percent of these cases were reported in Monrovia and other parts of Montserrado County.[29,30] It was customary to isolate all suspect cases in one area of the ETU; if confirmed positive, cases were then moved to the more restricted area for Ebola positive cases. This meant that patients testing negative could have been directly exposed to infected Ebola cases. This would make them contacts at risk for Ebola infection within twenty-one days after release from the ETU. Given the nonexistent referral system at the time, the risks were even greater. In addition, Ebola survivors also needed care, as many people manifested symptoms or presented with illnesses requiring care in a regular hospital setting and not an ETU with all the clinical demands and restrictions on staff.

When the government decided to cremate the corpses of everyone who died during the height of the epidemic, MSF provided two incinerators for the crematorium and safely removed corpses in body bags (spraying and double bagging the bodies inside the individual room as per EVD protocol) from the ETU to the crematorium. The rooms were subsequently sprayed with 0.5% chlorine after the bodies were removed.[28]

In October, Médecins Sans Frontières France (MSF-F), another MSF operational center, arrived in Monrovia to supplement the activities of MSF-Belgium. At the time of their arrival, response activities were intensifying, and most health care workers were still afraid to go to work. Health workers who remained were directly engaged in some aspect of the response or assigned to work in the ETU. Consequently, routine health care services were severely compromised. Patients with acute and chronic illnesses unrelated to Ebola were unable to get the care and treatment they needed, especially if they required hospitalization. Left untreated, many may have died unnecessarily during the peak of the epidemic, in numbers higher than we will ever know. The entire health care delivery system collapsed. Hospitals in Monrovia were operating at 5%, and outpatient facilities were operating at 50% with a lot of limitations.[28,31]

MSF France's inpatient facility was put in place and renovated. The response priorities began to shift, and the focus turned to providing care for patients with acute and chronic illness unrelated to Ebola. Patients suspected of having Ebola who tested negative within the seventy-two-hour isolation period were discharged from ETUs for Ebola survivors. Restoration of routine health services was more seriously being addressed. Creating designated isolation units in hospitals or other secondary health facilities and training staff fit for purpose became a part of the conversation. Infection prevention and control was often highlighted as a means of protecting the clinical staff and the patient from Ebola. In this light, MSF France proposed to the Ministry of Health that an inpatient referral health care facility be opened to address these needs. They suggested that this could make people more inclined to develop better "health-seeking behavior" and "regain . . . confidence in the health system."[32]

Patients were classified into two categories: (1) convalescent Ebola patients requiring hospitalization after discharge (EVD negative) from hospitalization at an ETC and (2) suspected Ebola patients with a negative test seventy-two hours after the onset of symptoms. Setting up the facility was pivotal, as it built confidence for people to return to normal and routine health services.

United Nations Mission for Ebola Emergency Response

The United Nations Mission for Ebola Emergency Response (UNMEER) was established on September 19, by a resolution of the UN General Assembly and adopted by the Security Council, to mount a coordinated, unified, and multinational effort in response to the Ebola outbreak in West Africa.[33,34,35]

The creation of UNMEER was primed by a report presented to international partners by the IMS team, detailing the status of the outbreak, and by WHO Director-General Margaret Chan's situation report to UN Secretary-General Ban Ki-moon and other UN officials (including Dr. Bruce Aylward, Dr. David Nabarro, Mr. Peter Graaf, and Dr. Alex Gasasira). Director-General Chan's report stated that the "full capacities of the United Nations be brought to bear under a unified coordination mechanism" if the epidemic was to be effectively contained. By then, the WHO had declared a "public health emergency of international concern" and the epidemic had reached unparalleled proportions in the Mano River Union (Guinea, Liberia, and Sierra Leone). In view of the gravity of Director-General Chan's situation report, Secretary-General Ban set up UNMEER, a mission designed to respond unequivocally to the Ebola epidemic in West Africa. It was stipulated that this mission would be dissolved when the crisis ended and the Ebola virus disease was no longer a threat to the region. Dr. David Nabarro was named the special envoy to the secretary-general on Ebola.[36]

The establishment of UNMEER and the expanded roles of the US military and CDC were force-multipliers in the situation. These entities brought invaluable expertise, personnel, and funding. Their presence had a psychological effect, as people started to trust the Liberian government's messages.

UNICEF

UNICEF provided safe drinking water, psychosocial support, education, child protective services, and nutrition assistance. They also improved sanitation and hygiene by promoting infection prevention and control. In 2014, UNICEF shipped 68 metric tons of urgently needed health and hygiene supplies from its global supply hub in Copenhagen, Denmark. The consignment included basic emergency items for frontline health workers:[37] personal protective equipment and chlorine; 450,000 pairs of latex gloves;[35] 27 metric tons of concentrated chlorine for disinfection and water purification; intravenous fluids, oral rehydration salts, and ready-to-use therapeutic food to feed patients undergoing treatment; water, sanitation, and hygiene (WASH) equipment to support infection control; and motorcycles and other logistical support to enable community health workers and other partners to move more freely around the communities.[37] UNICEF deployed teams of traditional communicators to spread prevention messaging across Liberia and produced print communications and radio programming to raise public awareness of the outbreak.

Supplies were distributed to health facilities nationwide, many of which were critically short of basic health care materials. I worked with Sheldon Yett, then country representative of UNICEF Liberia. We were extremely grateful for these supplies, which helped us to begin disinfecting, resupplying, and reopening clinics and hospitals so that essential health services could resume.

At the turning over ceremony—when the supplies were delivered and presented before the local community—Yett said, "Basic health care cannot be Ebola's next casualty. UNICEF has been working on multiple fronts since the beginning of the outbreak to provide critically needed supplies as well arming communities with the information they need to stop the spread of the disease. This shipment will complement those efforts with a new surge of supplies to equip health facilities, support infection control, and protect health workers on the front lines."[37]

Yett told me that the supplies were procured and delivered with support from USAID's Ebola Disaster Assistance Response Team, which was coordinating US government efforts. At the turning over ceremony, Tim Callaghan, USAID Ebola Disaster Assistance Response Team leader, also said, "We are facing the most devastating Ebola outbreak in history. It will take a coordinated global effort to bring this under control. For months, we have been working with UNICEF to ensure that medical equipment and critical messages are getting to the people and places that need it most."[37]

From October, the UN Office of Project Services (UNOPS) partnered with the WHO, with support from the Bill & Melinda Gates Foundation, to procure nineteen additional ambulances. UNOPS worked closely with the IMS and MOHSW during the recovery phase in building a resilient health system by rehabilitating existing health infrastructure, building triages, and improving waste management systems.

European Union

The European Union (EU) provided financial support, technical experts, and other personnel from member countries. It closely monitored the progression of the Ebola outbreak through its Emergency Response Coordination Centre, collaborating with the European Centre for Disease Prevention and Control, the EU member states' health authorities, WHO, and other international organizations. From March 2014, the European Commission had been scaling up its response. On August 15, the Council of the European Union called for a strong follow-up and a coordinated international response to the Ebola outbreak.[38] A total of €147 million (US$157 million) was pledged initially, plus €3.9 million (US$4.2 million) of humanitarian aid, followed by a global package of €140.5 million (US$149.6 million), as of September 9, 2014.[38] The monies pledged were earmarked for designated systems or programs: €3 million (US$3.2 million) went to ASEOWA. Health care systems received €38m (US$40.5 million) to reinforce and bring humanitarian assistance and €5 million (US$5.3 million) to provide and support mobile laboratories. The governments of Liberia (€50.5 million, or US$53.8 million) and Sierra Leone (€47 million, or US$50 million) received a total of €97.5 million (US$104 million) to deliver improved public services and maintain economic and political stability.[38] The European Civil Protection and Humanitarian Aid Operations (ECHO) deployed humanitarian specialists to link with onsite partners (primarily MSF Belgium and MSF France, WHO, and the International Federation of Red Cross and Red Crescent Societies) and local authorities.[38] Individual member countries also sent specialized teams and organizations to provide technical assistance.

Government of the People's Republic of China

The government of the People's Republic of China brought in the first plane load of a large number of medical supplies and equipment, medics, military personnel, and logistics to set up an ETU. Like many other countries in the Ebola response, this was the first time China was actively engaged in responding to a public health crisis off its shores. Interacting was quite an experience for them and for us, in part due to the language barriers. None of the Liberians spoke Chinese and few of the Chinese contingent spoke English fluently. Consequently, most of our communication was through an interpreter. Nonetheless, we got along very well together.

One meeting, on November 14, brought together the US and Chinese CDC delegations. Both teams had met previously in other settings and were quite familiar with each other. To our relief, the mood in the room was cordial and somewhat relaxed. Considering the global tension between Beijing and Washington, we were surprised that the two teams worked together harmoniously. Perhaps it was in the interest of global health security, each being cognizant of the fact that diseases have no boundaries, transcending politics and trade wars.

The Chinese came with a clear mission, which they executed rapidly. A few days after their arrival, they began construction of a 100-bed Ebola treatment center, at the Samuel Kanyon Doe (SKD) Sports Complex, meeting the highest standards required for infectious disease control and prevention hospitals, covering a land mass of more than 20,000 square meters.[39] China dispatched 500 medical personnel in three batches to Liberia to work in every capacity in managing Ebola. Chinese Ambassador Zhang Yue and Liberian Minister of Foreign Affairs Augustine Kpehe Ngafuan signed two agreements on the projects of building and operating an ETU and providing anti-Ebola material. The ETU was valued around US$41 million.[39]

It was fascinating to watch their operations. The Chinese were disciplined, respectful, and very efficient. The China ETU project was launched on October 26 and was in full operation on November 25. It was one of Liberia's best treatment centers at that critical time in our history. On November 15, a 163-member medical team, comprising military personnel from the Chinese Liberation Army, arrived in Monrovia via China Air.[39] The Chinese medical team was headed by Wang Yungui, who was also the vice president of the Third Medical Military University of China. He emphasized China's determination in helping Liberia and other Ebola affected countries.[40] They operated the center in typical hierarchical fashion of a military operation. On January 12, 2015, the first three surviving Ebola patients were discharged from the China ETU (or SKD 1, as it was also called). The Chinese medical team invited the Liberian team to witness the discharge protocol. Our team, including case management team lead Dr. Moses Massaquoi, were able to observe treatment, care, and discharge procedures and attend a special ceremony for the three Ebola survivors, officially and publicly acknowledging their survival and discharge. It was indeed a magnificent day, seeing an eight-year-old boy and two young women who had survived Ebola and were well enough to go home. The ceremony was highlighted by a tree planting ceremony, where each survivor planted a tree. There was also a palm printing, with a specialized red ink to mark the date of their recovery and discharge. A band played, refreshments were served, and each survivor was given gifts to restart their lives. There was a lot of goodwill. One woman received a scholarship to travel to China to perfect her skills in table tennis.

China's generosity to the response was motivated by two factors: first, to prevent EVD from reaching its shores and second, "to pursue soft power in Africa." China's financial contribution toward EVD control in West Africa was "much more impressive when adjusted for gross domestic product (GDP) per capita," even if outmatched by the United States and EU countries. Ebola presented an opportunity for China to expand its global health governance, become directly involved in a global epidemic response, and diversify its humanitarian engagement.[41]

According to senior Chinese health officials, providing aid to West Africa was crucial in China's efforts to construct a "barrier" against the spread of the virus. Minister Li Bin of the National Health and Family Planning Commission of the People's Republic of China (NHFPC) was candid when she explained why China supported West Africa's fight against Ebola: "Infectious diseases know no boundaries. . . . China, by helping West African nations, is also helping itself."[39] Overall, China responded to the Ebola epidemic in West Africa with unprecedented generosity. While it was not unusual for China to offer humanitarian aid to countries affected by natural disasters, this was the first time China extended massive humanitarian aid to countries fighting a public health emergency. By late November 2014, China had—throughout four consecutive phases, in April, August, September, and October— offered US$123 million (750 million yuan) worth of humanitarian aid to the global Ebola control efforts, China's largest-ever response to an international humanitarian crisis.[39] The package included the provision of in-kind contributions comprising ambulances, motorcycles, medical equipment, prevention care supplies, food aid, and deployment of medical teams and public health experts, as well as labs and treatment centers. WHO Director-General Margaret Chan called China's commitment "a huge boost, morally and operationally."[41]

Government of the Republic of Cuba

In September 2014, the United Nations and its specialized agency, the World Health Organization (WHO), issued a call for medical collaboration in response to the medical crisis and social disaster caused by the Ebola virus epidemic in West Africa. The Cuban ambassador to Liberia, H. E. Jorge Lefebre Nicolo, said, "We are ready 100% to collaborate with the Americans. We should fight against Ebola and anything else should be put aside. We cannot see our brothers from Africa in difficult times."[42,43]

Cuban authorities responded immediately to the call by offering specialized help for the epidemic, in collaboration with WHO. A group of 256 Cuban doctors, nurses, and other health professionals provided direct care during the Ebola epidemic in Sierra Leone, Liberia, and Guinea from October 2014 to April 2015. Enrique Beldarraín Chaple, chief of the research department at the Cuban National Information Centre of Sciences, said, "The response of the Cuban medical teams to the Ebola epidemic in West Africa is only one example of the Cuban efforts to strengthening health care provision in areas of need throughout the world."[42,43] Cuban health authorities offered a group of doctors the chance to volunteer for the risky work of treating the disease in West Africa. In the three countries, they attended to 1,728 patients and saved an estimated 356 people from death due to the disease. Two Cuban volunteers died during their tour of duty, both from malaria. Only one Cuban volunteer became infected with Ebola, a forty-three-year-old specialist in internal medicine who worked with patients in Sierra Leone. He was treated in Switzerland, returned to Cuba for a recovery period, and subsequently returned to Sierra Leone to continue his work in Ebola treatment.

The Cuban commitment to international medical collaboration is a model that could be more widely applied. A group of doctors belonging to the Henry Reeve Contingent were identified by the Cuban health authorities and offered the chance to volunteer in West Africa. Those who accepted received the first part of their training in Cuba at the Institute of Tropical Medicine Pedro Kouri facility. This training center was established for the training of health personnel in the treatment and control of disease, with simulations of different risk scenarios. Training included management and biosecurity standards for handling Ebola patients, the use of special protective suits to be worn during contact with the sick, mounting field hospitals, and a range of treatments and diagnostic techniques to be used. They were also updated on the clinical, epidemiologic, and diagnostic aspects of the condition. These courses and seminars were given by prominent professors of different specialties, such as internal medicine, emergency and critical care medicine, epidemiology, microbiology, clinical laboratory, and nursing care. Medical staff then received a second intensive training in Liberia in the red zone, with patients suffering from Ebola. The last subgroup completed training on November 23, 2014; all were certified by WHO to serve in the Ebola treatment unit.

The New Ministry of Defense that was being built in the 1980s by President Samuel Doe was used as the location for an ETU. In mid-August that ground was covered with grass. It was one of the sites that President Sirleaf, Ambassador Malac, and I identified as a suitable site to build an ETU. WHO, in partnership with US government agencies in Liberia, began the construction of the ETU, which was built in a short time by soldiers of the US Army and named MOD1. Cuban professionals were assigned to work in MOD1. The facility doctors were aided by Liberian and African Union health workers from Rwanda, Uganda, Ethiopia, Namibia, and Angola, all temporarily employed by the WHO.

Dr. James Soka Moses, a Liberian physician, was head of the MOD1 clinical team. At the height of the outbreak, Dr. Moses took on one of the toughest jobs in the country, working in one of Monrovia's largest ETUs, managing a high-volume, highly contagious patient population while adopting a collaborative, systems-based public health approach. Once Ebola transmissions reduced, he turned his focus to Liberia's thousands of survivors through the Ebola Survivor's Clinic, providing treatment, support, and training for patients and leading an important program to mitigate sexual transmission of the disease. In 2017,

Dr. Moses was featured in the CNN documentary *Unseen Enemy*, which recounts the effects of the Ebola, SARS, and Zika outbreaks, as well as the consequences of emerging infectious disease threats on global health security.[44]

The Cuban leadership demonstrated a remarkable level of global solidarity in health with their response to the Ebola epidemic in West Africa. Cuban health professionals provided admirable support for direct care of the affected population under extremely difficult conditions, demonstrating great discipline and cohesiveness as a group. These efforts mirrored the remarkable success of the Cuban domestic health program in bringing about high levels of health care despite challenging economic conditions.

Germany

Chancellor Angela Merkel announced on September 17, 2014, Germany's intention to provide logistical support to Liberia.[45,46] Her government sent transport planes as well as a standby aircraft to fly medical staff out of infected countries for treatment. The Germans also sent a mobile hospital and helped built an ETU. This was in response to a letter from President Sirleaf to numerous heads of governments, asking for help. Merkel's office said the chancellor had been "very moved" by the request. "The situation is dramatic," said Merkel. "We will act very quickly and will be available with everything that we have at our disposal. We will meet our responsibilities."[43,44]

For example, there was a substantial need to conceive and construct a facility that met the epidemiological situation at that time: one suitable for diagnosis and treatment of other relevant infectious diseases, in the context of an ongoing Ebola outbreak. The pilot project of a Severe Infection Temporary Treatment Unit (SITTU) was launched. In conventional ETUs, patients were separated according to their risk of being infected by Ebola virus. In the SITTU design, patients were separated by their probability of not being infected by Ebola virus: suspect cases (any patient presenting and fulfilling case definition criteria); unlikely cases (patients with one negative Ebola polymerase chain reaction [PCR] result after admission); and confirmed negative cases (patients testing negative for EVD twice, forty-eight hours apart). This was the situation in Liberia when on December 23, the ETU SKD2, located at the Samuel Kanyon Doe (SKD) Sports Complex in Monrovia, became operational. The Chinese had constructed SKD1 on the opposite side of the stadium.

The large size of the SKD2 facility and increased facility quality requirements commissioned by national and intergovernmental stakeholders proved to be a challenge for the speed at which SKD2 became operational. Coupled with setbacks during the construction period due to delayed delivery of building materials (e.g., a high-temperature incinerator) and delivery of broken materials (e.g., sewer pipes), the construction time for the installation was about four months. This ETU was designed as a WHO standard 100-bed ETU and was supported by the German government with deployment of material and staff from the German Red Cross and the German Armed Forces. By the end of December 2014 there were more than 1,000 ETU beds available countrywide, while the number of hospitalized suspected Ebola cases had fallen to below 100 in the entire country. Due to persistent fear of Ebola, many patients with non-EVD infectious diseases were not admitted to ordinary health care facilities as these facilities were not prepared or equipped to manage potentially highly contagious patients.[47]

World Bank

The World Bank's role in the Ebola response was pivotal. The outbreak was clearly exacerbated by countries already under stress. In Liberia, the country's health system was still recovering from the ravage of over fourteen years of civil war. Although Liberia's economy was one of the fastest growing prior to the epidemic, there remained high levels of poverty with poor road infrastructure, limited access to safe water, unreliable power, and undependable communications networks. There were severe shortages of health workers, health facilities, pharmaceuticals, and other necessary materials, as well as funds to pay health workers. In the year before the outbreak, there had been four strikes by workers in the public health sector due to the inability of the government to pay required wages, put workers on government payroll, or provide appropriate housing for those sent to posts in rural areas. Health workers generally had little confidence in the system and did not trust health authorities. Given the high level of suspicion people had of the government in a post-conflict environment and the government's inability to provide health services and safely handle dead bodies as EVD cases escalated, a vicious cycle of suspicion, miscommunication, mistrust, exposure to infectious dead bodies, and explosive transmission took hold.[48]

The issue of hazard pay became paramount. People working in the treatment units were requesting hazard payment and death benefits in case they got infected with Ebola. I was part of the negotiation between the ministries of health and finance, the Liberia Medical and Dental Council, and the Health Workers Association of Liberia. At that meeting, Finance Minister Amara Konneh signed an agreement with the workers on a salary scale that was agreed upon by all parties. The World Bank Group Ebola Emergency Response Project (EERP) was instrumental in filling this gap, according to Amara Konneh.

On September 16, 2014, the World Bank approved EERP to support the governments of Guinea, Liberia, and Sierra Leone, contributing in the short term to the control of the Ebola epidemic. The World Bank Group's Board of Executive Directors "approved a US$285 million grant to finance Ebola-containment efforts underway in Guinea, Liberia and Sierra Leone, as well as to help communities in the three countries cope with the socioeconomic impact of the crisis and, rebuild and strengthen essential health services."[49] The grant was part of the nearly US$1 billion previously announced by the World Bank Group (WBG) for these countries hardest hit by the Ebola crisis.[49] The group's president reiterated the international communities' call to support our efforts in Liberia, for which we were extremely grateful. This additional financing would address the critical needs of affected countries and assist in intensifying our efforts in halting Ebola. Jim Yong Kim, WBG president said, "This deadly outbreak is far from over, and the international community must continue to do everything we can to support these countries until we get to zero cases."[49] The grant provided additional financing to the Ebola Emergency Response Project that was approved by the WBG's Board on September 16, 2014, including US$72 million for Guinea, US$115 million for Liberia, and US$98 million for Sierra Leone, the three countries most affected by Ebola.[49]

EERP financed essential supplies and staffing of the Ebola treatment units (ETUs), personal protection equipment (PPE), and hazard pay and death benefits for Ebola caregivers and other health workers providing essential health services for non-Ebola conditions. It also financed safe and dignified burials, it provided support for contact tracing, social mobilization, provision of food, and other essential services to communities affected and quarantined due to Ebola exposure. EERP totaled US$390 million, consisting of an original International Development Association (IDA) grant (US$105 million) and an additional financing grant (US$285 million) from the Bank's Crisis Response Window. The original IDA grant was approved on September 16, 2014; the additional financing was approved on November 18.[50]

In March 2015, a meeting was held in Brussels, attended by the presidents of Guinea, Liberia, and Sierra Leone. These leaders humbly asked for help from donors to repair the damage to their economies as the epidemic began to wane. They expressed their confidence that they were winning the public health battle and had to remain focused on stamping out new infections. By then, around 10,000 people had died of Ebola cumulatively in the three countries. Each faced severe setbacks to their economies, which had previously been performing relatively well. "Victory against the virus is in sight but we must guard against complacency. There will not be total victory until we get to a resilient zero [new cases] in the three most affected countries," Sierra Leone's president, Ernest Bai Koroma, told the conference. Ebola cases had declined sharply in recent weeks, but a recent surge in new infections in Sierra Leone was concerning. "It's easier to go from 100 [cases] to 10 than from 10 to zero," Guinea's president, Alpha Condé, said.

At that time, according to EU officials, international donors had pledged nearly US$5 billion to help combat the Ebola epidemic, although only about half of that money had been disbursed to affected countries. Schools, farms, and markets closed during the outbreak, casting a chill on business as investors left and government finances weakened. A fall in global commodity prices compounded the region's problems. The World Bank estimated the epidemic would cost the three countries at least US$1.6 billion in lost economic growth in 2015, or more than 12% of their combined output. President Sirleaf said the three countries believed a regional approach to recovery was best. "This can only be achieved with your support," she told the conference, which brought together 600 delegates from around the world. "There is no doubt this will require significant resources, perhaps even a Marshall plan," she said, referring to the large US aid program to rebuild Europe after World War II. President Sirleaf mentioned that the three Mano River Union nations intended to draft a regional recovery plan to present to the International Monetary Fund and the World Bank at their meetings in April. They were not expecting new aid pledges at the Brussels conference. Sierra Leone President Koroma wanted debt relief, grants, and concessionary loans and was seeking support to rebuild social services and to revitalize the private sector.[51] Whether or not his desire for debt relief was to crystallize is something else for another day.

World Food Programme

The World Food Programme (WFP) played an essential role in the response to the outbreak by providing extensive common logistics services to all responders through the Regional Special Operation 200773.[52] Under this operation, "Logistics and Capacity Development Support for the Humanitarian Community's Response to the Ebola Virus Disease Outbreak in Liberia," WFP set up the logistics backbone of the health response across the three countries.[52] WFP also extended the provision of adequate logistics support through June 2016 during the health system recovery phase, as well as storage and transport services of personal protection equipment and infection prevention and control kits for international organizations and the MOH.

Through its special operation, WFP provided uninterrupted logistics response capacity, including transporting and storing cargo, ensuring the national government had the necessary assets and capacity to respond timely and efficiently to other potential EVD outbreaks and other non-health emergencies in Liberia. WFP also provided its exit strategy for when the outbreak ended, to facilitate the government's transition from response to recovery. In addition, WFP provided a tailored and nimble level of logistics support to mandated national entities and health partners, such as the WHO, free of charge until June 2016. The support included, among other things, the continued operability of main logistics bases, forward logistics bases, targeted transport services, and logistics coordination when required. Last-mile transportation was necessary for WFP support to the counties' health teams either by air, road, or sea. The government of Liberia in 2015 jointly designed a transition strategy that enabled WFP to hand over logistics storage facilities to the General Services Agency (GSA) headed by Mary Broh. Once handed over, the facilities were managed by government of Liberia institutions (GSA and MOH) to ensure continuous operability and sustainability. The logistics structure helped with building the resilient health services and rebuilding clinics and hospitals; it also helped with IPC supplies to facilities once a new minister of health was appointed in 2015. The logistics system offered an opportunity for improvement of Liberia's Emergency Preparedness and Response capacity, in line with the government's commitment and government acknowledgment of the importance of disaster preparedness and response.

Media

The Ministry of Information, Cultural Affairs, and Tourism (MICAT), headed by Minister Lewis Brown, was the umbrella under which all media (Liberian and international) functioned. Adulai Kamara (now deceased) coordinated local independent media. Jana Telfer, communications officer for CDC, transcribed major themes from IMS meetings for the mass media. There were press briefings, weekly, often daily, held by the minister, along with his deputies, to which the press corps was invited. Minister Brown presented the government's position on the response. The government did not want information on the response being disseminated from multiple sources, so I attended these briefings to give details on IMS response activities and updates on case load, ETUs, and general information. There was always a question-and-answer period at the end of the briefings. I granted many interviews to the BBC through its Liberia correspondent, Jonathan Paye-layleh, CNN, Radio France Internationale, Voice of America, Al Jazeera, the *New York Times*, and others. I also gave regular updates on the national radio station, ELBC, Truth FM radio and community radio stations across the country. Similar updates were given to local print and electronic media: Front Page Africa, The Daily Observer, and New Democrat.

The Social Mobilization pillar had several working groups: Media Support and Documentation (MSD) Partner Working Group and Messages and Materials Development (MMD) Partner Working Group. The purpose of the MSD was to develop and implement various approaches to supplement the MOHSW efforts; gather public health messages, news releases, and other information produced by partner organizations, to identify commonalities, differences, and gaps in messaging; monitor news reports, compiling messages and trends, and sharing summary information promptly and effectively; gather information about partner plans and actions; and conduct analysis of news reports to identify disparities and alignments in health messaging. In theory, this working group was responsible for establishing and maintaining collaboration and information-sharing methods with MMD on regular reports of news analysis, identification of trends, and identification of misinformation, and with the Social Mobilization team, through weekly reports, summarizing findings from the previous week, and outreach to member partners as circumstances indicated. However, because a similar or duplicative group existed within MICAT, the two groups were later merged and housed there.

The objectives of this group were to support the development of briefings and media coverage to a broad national communication strategy that linked MOHSW and partner messages and actions to public and intragovernmental outreach activities, facilitated by the Ministry of Information, Cultural Affairs, and Tourism; coordinate harmonization among government and partner media and other public messaging related to public health aspects of the national Ebola response; and monitor news reports and identify issues and trends to assist in supporting development of new media and social mobilization messages.

The purpose of MMD was to develop, field test, and revise or update key messages for use in posters, training packages (for such audiences as community health volunteers or teachers), pictorial contents, radio jingles, announcements, and videos. One of the key products of this working group was the Ebola Message Guide, which was revised regularly to reflect new knowledge and the changing landscape. The objectives of the MMD Partner Working Group were to develop messages and educational materials to promote and inform the public and other targeted audiences on Ebola prevention, response activation, home protection, community care, and risk behaviors; ensure that messages were audience-specific, gender-focused, and culturally and contextually relevant; design messages appropriate to the channel of distribution; and ensure that messages were responsive to rumor, concern, rapid change, and new developments within the response.

Nongovernmental Organizations and Private Educational Institutions

Local and international nongovernmental organizations (NGOs) were engaged in several active response elements: case management; cross-border screening; social mobilization; community engagement; safe and dignified burials; water, sanitation, and hygiene (WASH); and nutrition services.

Africare performed contact tracing, community education, and distribution of chlorine and buckets with hygiene promotion at public places.

Angie Brooks Randell, a local civil society organization, championed women and children's health.

CARE International held community meetings, directed and incentivized house-to-house mobilization, provided cell phones and bicycles for GCHVs and some community leaders, and performed contact tracing, community education, and distribution of chlorine and buckets with hygiene promotion at public places.

Carter Center directed training of trainers (TOT) training, engaged community leaders, supported mental health clinicians, and engaged the National Council of Chiefs and Elders.

Clinton Health Access Initiative (CHAI) Country Director Dr. Moses Massaquoi headed the Case Management pillar. His deputy, Lauren Zinner, and her staff supported the logistics arm of the response and managed the supply chain system. Former US president Bill Clinton visited Liberia in May 2015, during the epidemic.

Gbowee Peace Foundation Africa (GPFA), founded by Leymah Gbowee, a Liberian and 2011 Nobel Peace Prize laureate, mobilized twelve community-based organizations (CBOs) and four news reporters in Monrovia and news in rural areas. Through the GPFA Ebola Outreach Awareness Initiative (GEOAI), it provided small grants, promoted awareness, and provided training on Ebola prevention through a partnership with the MOHSW Division of Disease Prevention and Control. GPFA disseminated Ebola fact sheets and posters; it supported thirty-five groups in phase two, including nine local CBOs, nine rural groups, seven rural radio stations, and nine news reporters.

International Organization for Migration (IOM) assisted with cross-border activities and screening at points of entry, training, development and provision of materials, radio production and airing, dissemination of print materials (posters, etc.), and community meetings.

International Rescue Committee (IRC) supported community-based initiatives.

Johns Hopkins Center for Communication Programs (CCP) provided technical support to the division of health programs and community network support and helped create awareness of Ebola.

Last Mile Health helped with planning and strategy development, partner coordination, and research (KAP, focus groups, interviews, field testing); disseminated print materials (posters, etc.); directed TOT trainings; trained frontline mobilizers; and supported community meetings.

Liberia Crusaders for Peace assisted with planning and strategy development, partner coordination, development of materials (IEC and training materials), radio production and airing, print materials dissemination (posters, etc.), training of trainers, direct training of frontline mobilizers, journalist/media trainings, community meetings, house-to-house mobilization, engagement of community leaders, community drama/theater and storytelling, and community announcements and town criers.

Liberia National Red Cross Society (LNRCS) handled dead body management. It ran community meetings; performed house-to-house mobilization; engaged community leaders; provided logistical support, vehicles, and training for burial teams; and trained burial teams and contact tracers.

Medical Emergency Relief International (MERCI), a prominent local NGO, provided community and grassroots services in Montserrado, Maryland, and River Gee Counties.

Medical Teams International (MTI) ran ETUs in Margibi and Bong Counties, disseminated print materials (posters, etc.), ran training of trainers (TOT), trained frontline mobilizers, and mobilized community meetings through house-to-house outreach.

Mercy Corps established an army of community mobilizers across Liberia and carried out social mobilization and awareness services.

Samaritan's Purse provided initial support by running a treatment unit in Lofa and Monrovia. But when its staff got infected with Ebola, it pulled out and left the country. When Samaritan's Purse returned to Liberia, it started supporting direct training of frontline mobilizers and distributed Ebola prevention materials with community awareness prevention messaging.

Save the Children provided psychosocial support to families and children who were infected by the Ebola virus.

Search for Common Ground (SFCG) Liberia is comprised of twenty Liberian civil society groups working as a united front educating communities in seven target counties. Supported by Action Aid, OSIWA, and Medica Mondiale, SFCG helped with interpersonal communications and door-to-door outreach in target communities, worked closely with existing community structure to achieve their objectives, and assisted with house-to-house mobilization and engagement of community leaders.

Tony Blair Africa Governance Initiative (now Tony Blair Institute for Global Change) provided support to PACE, the incident management system team, and the Social Mobilization pillar. The foundation provided support in coordination, media relations, and community mobilization.

Welthungerhilfe assisted with planning and strategy development, partner coordination, research (KAP, focus groups, interviews, field testing), development of materials (IEC and training materials), radio production and airing, print material dissemination (posters, etc.), printing (books and special aids for children and youth), TOT trainings, direct training of frontline mobilizers, engagement of community leaders, community drama/theater and storytelling, community care, and training government partners.

Recovery, Rebuilding, and Resiliency

On May 9, 2015, WHO declared Liberia free of Ebola virus disease in human-to-human transmission for the first time since the outbreak began in March 2014, and forty-two days after the March 28 burial of the last person with a laboratory-confirmed positive Ebola test. In the declaration, WHO acknowledged that interruption of transmission was a monumental achievement for a country that had reported the highest number of deaths in the largest, longest, and most complex outbreak since Ebola first emerged in 1976.[1]

Jubilation filled the streets nationwide, particularly in Monrovia, where an official ceremony to celebrate this milestone was held on May 11 at the Centennial Pavilion, the main government venue for state celebrations. The ceremony was attended by all branches of the government. President Sirleaf led the way, followed by Vice President Joseph Boakai; the speaker of the house of representatives, the Honorable Alex Tyler; Chief Justice Francis Kporkpoh; cabinet ministers; members of the legislature; and foreign dignitaries. President Faure Gnassingbé of Togo, who was appointed the coordinator of the West African Ebola response, attended, representing ECOWAS. Honorable Hanna Serwaa Tetteh, Ghana's minister of foreign affairs and regional integration, represented her president, President John Dramani Mahama. It was a great day in Liberia. At last, we believed then, we had our freedom from Ebola.

While WHO was confident that Liberia had interrupted transmission, outbreaks persisted in neighboring Guinea and Sierra Leone, creating a high risk that infected people might cross into Liberia through the region's exceptionally porous borders. The government was fully aware of the need to remain on high alert and had the experience, capacity, and support from international partners to do so.

There were three subsequent, though smaller, Ebola flare-ups, in June and November 2015 and in March and April 2016. The national response to the reemergence rapidly and effectively interrupted transmission, a testament to the improvement in the government's capacity to understand epidemiological trends and manage outbreaks. After two negative tests for Ebola virus disease, forty-two days (twenty-one-day incubation cycles of the virus times two) after the last patient was confirmed positive in Liberia, on January 14, 2016, WHO again declared Liberia free of Ebola in the human population. All three affected countries now had no new cases. Sierra Leone and Guinea had both been declared free of Ebola on November 7, and December 29, 2015, respectively.[2] Liberia's final Ebola-free declaration was on June 1, 2016, following the March outbreak.[1] WHO and CDC maintained an enhanced presence in Liberia until the end of 2016, as the response transitioned from outbreak control to active surveillance for new or imported cases, and into the beginning of the recovery of essential health services. During this period, CDC opened its first country office in Liberia, with Dr. Desmond Williams as the country director.

The EVD outbreak had major effects on health services, which led to significant declines in utilization of health services from August to December 2014, compared to the same period in 2012 and 2013. These declines were partly due to temporary closures of health facilities and partly because of lower attendance due to the community's distrust of the health system. Those who made it to health facilities were often shunned and therefore refused to go; even women in active labor refused to seek care at public health facilities, many of whom died in the process. The fear of Ebola simply made matters worse.[3]

With limited access to public sector health facilities, where prior to the Ebola epidemic services had been provided free, out-of-pocket spending increased due to the public use of alternative services, further limiting access to care. The resultant increased morbidity and mortality reversed gains that had been made earlier. Outpatient department (OPD) visits fell by 61% for Liberia, and 51% if Montserrado County is excluded.[3] The declines in OPD attendance were observed in all counties and were greatest in Montserrado, Margibi, Bomi, and Grand Cape Mount Counties.[3] These were also the counties with the highest cumulative EVD cases. Similar reductions were observed in reproductive, maternal, newborn and child health services, and immunization attendance. The declines in the first antenatal care visit, in hospital deliveries, measles, and DTP3 vaccinations were slightly smaller than for OPD visits: 43%, 38%, 45%, and 53%, respectively.[3] The largest reduction was observed in August 2014. However, measles vaccinations increased considerably in December as a result of an accelerated campaign.[3]

As the outbreak waned, immense efforts were necessary to reduce EVD cases to zero and sustain it. At the same time, efforts toward restoring normal routine health services had to be robust. These efforts were led by Dr. Bernice Dahn, then minister of health, and her deputy minister for planning, research and policy, Yah Zolia. This transition had to be different from Liberia's previous approach to delivering health services—it had to incorporate the lessons learned during the outbreak. Various recommendations were drawn from assessments undertaken by the MOHSW, WHO, and other collaborating partners (UNDP, USAID, UNICEF, and others). How would we, as a country, stamp out this epidemic, transition toward restoration of health services, and rebuild our health system in a resilient manner? The goal was that the system would be equipped to deliver better, more effective, and sustainable health services, while managing any future shocks or health threats. Fundamentally, the MOHSW wanted to restore the gains lost due to the EVD crisis and provide health security for the people of Liberia. The ministry's intent was to accelerate progress toward universal health coverage by improving access to safe and quality health services, with a strong emergency management system. The MOHSW knew that the public trust in the government's ability to provide adequate and effective health services had to be restored.

The ministry had scheduled a review of the National Health Policy and Plan (2011–2021) for October 2014. However, the eruption of EVD interrupted this process. A consultation on the process for the review was held on November 19 with the Health Sector Coordination Committee (HSCC), which gave its conditional approval. The HSCC is the highest decision-making body of the health sector and is comprised of government ministries and agencies, UN agencies involved in health care, donors, and the private sector.[3]

On December 10 and 11, WHO, the West African Health Organization (WAHO), the World Bank, and the European Union met in Geneva with high-level delegations from the EVD-affected West African countries. Key priorities were outlined at the meeting: strengthening the health workforce; enhancing community trust, engagement, and ownership; strengthening core public health capacities for surveillance and response; and ensuring predictable supplies and coordinated supply chains.[3]

Following the Geneva meeting, a National Consultative Stakeholders' meeting was held in Monrovia on January 12, 2015, to develop a concept note. On January 22, the concept note was presented to the president and her cabinet, which was approved. Preparations for the desk review and field assessments started immediately. Health system assessment guidelines, survey forms, and a questionnaire were developed, and teams of technical experts were trained to undertake a desk review (January and February) and field assessments (February) that would inform the development of an investment plan for rebuilding Liberia's health system.[3]

A MOHSW technical retreat was convened in Gbarnga, Bong County, March 25–27 to review and refine critical investment areas. During the retreat, an illustrative health system bottleneck analysis was undertaken to inform the prioritization of the strategic areas presented in the investment plan. Finally, a national stakeholder validation meeting was held April 6–8 to reach consensus on the investment plan. Agreed revisions proposed by county health teams, civil society, the private sector, regulators, legislators, other line ministries, and partners were incorporated into the final costed version of the investment plan.[3]

The Investment Plan for Building a Resilient Health System in Liberia outlined major weaknesses that preexisted or were exacerbated by the epidemic. The goal of the plan was to create a more resilient health system that could withstand any future shocks.[3] It recognized the weaknesses in training and skill sets of the existing health workforce, insufficiency in required numbers of trained staff per health facility, and gross deficiencies in health infrastructure nationally. It also recognized that laboratory and diagnostic services were not up to par. The same applied to the data and surveillance, health information, research, procurement, and supply chain systems. Pharmaceutical regulations, though on the books, were not strongly enforced. Sanitation services were either nonexistent or at a bare minimum, particularly in urban-rural interface and in shantytowns, where communities were not usually engaged, and personal health care expenditure was often extremely high.[3] All of these factors or weaknesses combined greatly impacted the health system as the epidemic spun out of control.

The investment plan priorities were aligned with existing priorities of the government, as defined in the National Health Policy and Plan (2011–2021),[3] as well as the Agenda for Transformation (AFT) and critical health sector priorities, agreed upon by the cabinet in early 2015.[4] The AFT "was the government of Liberia's five-year development strategy. It followed then, the Lift Liberia, Poverty Reduction Strategy (PRS), which professed to raise Liberia from post-conflict emergency reconstruction and positioned it for future growth."[4] The plan was tailored to the WHO framework that describes health systems in six core components or building blocks: "service delivery, health workforce, information, medical products, vaccines and technologies, financing, and leadership/governance."[5,6] The building blocks framework was noted to have potential gaps, as it ignored demand side (population), social determinants of health, facility-based and community-based services institutions, and societal partnerships with key stakeholders. All of these are within and outside of the health sector.[5] It doesn't present as a good "systems" diagram—it's not dynamic and points to only one direction, which is the health sector. The building blocks are interrelated, but they're not interdependent. In today's increasingly interconnected and interdependent world, where people, goods, and services move easily across borders, "it is more important than ever, to ensure that countries are able to respond in timely and effective fashion to contain, and indeed prevent, threats to public health."[7]

Consequently, the following investment areas were prioritized in the Investment Plan:

- Fit-for-purpose productive and motivated health workforce
- Reengineered health infrastructure
- Epidemic preparedness, surveillance, and response system
- Management capacity for medical supplies and diagnostics
- Enhancement of quality service delivery systems
- Comprehensive information, research, and communication management
- Sustainable community engagement
- Leadership and governance capacity
- Efficient health financing systems[3]

Because of the critical lessons learned from the outbreak, Liberia identified those nine priority investment areas for building a more resilient health system. Three additional priorities were aligned with the WHO building blocks: sustainable community engagement, reengineering of health infrastructure, and epidemic preparedness and response, including surveillance and the Early Warning, Alert and Response Network (EWARN).[3]

WHO's May 9, 2014, declaration that Liberia's human population was free of EVD also emphasized the importance of continued investment in surveillance, focusing on outbreak response capacity, risk communication, health promotion, and the Ebola vaccine, which was still in the developmental stage at that time.[2,8,9] Although community engagement and empowerment remained a high priority in health service provision, more support was needed to provide the necessary resources and proper collaboration to continue key activities, such as infection prevention and control, and emergency preparedness and response.[10]

In June, I was appointed deputy minister of health for disease surveillance and epidemic control, charged with implementing Liberia's epidemic preparedness and response, and expansion of the surveillance and EWARN to ensure the network was comprehensive enough to detect and respond to future health threats. In my new role, I was also assigned to: (1) establish a National Public Health Institute with a public health capacity-building component (the field epidemiology training program, or FETP); (2) establish functional emergency operations centers in each of Liberia's fifteen counties, as core structures for the stewardship and implementation of the WHO International Health Regulations of 2005; (3) revitalize and establish EWARN and Integrated Disease Surveillance and Response (IDSR) structures at national, county, district, and community levels; and (4) improve capacity for public health laboratories and establish a biobank.[3,11]

In August, Dr. Bernice Dahn, who was by then the minister of health, put me in charge of the establishment of the National Public Health Institute of Liberia (NPHIL). Senior ministry officials reviewed and discussed national public health institute (NPHI) core functions and developed an agenda for study tours to other countries with recognized NPHIs. The study tours were designed to learn from the experiences of well-established members of the International Association of National Public Health Institutes (IANPHI). Study tours were conducted to NPHIs in Thailand and Norway. I led the team of experts to Norway. Based on the positive outcomes from the study tours, the minister of health and the ministry's senior management team approved continued work toward the creation of NPHIL and consideration of whether or not it should be an autonomous agency of the government of Liberia.

We decided that the NPHIL would be a state-owned enterprise (SOE). SOEs are highly respected in Liberia because they can raise their own funding for sustainability and support socioeconomic programs. With substantive input from stakeholders, a one-year operational plan was finalized in February 2016 and used as the basis for establishing legislation for NPHIL. There were a series of workshops and stakeholders' meetings held in Gbarnga, Bong County; at Wulki Farms in Margibi County; then Buchanan, Grand Bassa County; Ganta, Nimba County; and in Montserrado County. At each of the stakeholders' meetings, international partners such as WHO, the CDC, and NIH were invited. They provided valuable input on what would become the architecture, strategic plan, and policy of NPHIL, which would be modeled after the US CDC. The NIH hired Ellen Cull, a strategic planning, management, and organizational consultant, to work with the Liberia team, as well as a team of experts from NIH's National Institute for Allergy and Infectious Diseases (NIAID), consisting of Dr. Anthony Fauci, director of NIAID, and Dr. H. Clifford Lane, NIAID's deputy director for clinical research. A week-long strategic planning session was held at the Golden Key Hotel in Monrovia. The US CDC dedicated an entire team led by Dr. Desmond Williams, then CDC country director, and a team of public health lawyers from its Center for Public Health Law Program, to work with the Liberian lawyers and drafting team. WHO also provided a consultant who traveled with the Liberia team to Norway and later visited Liberia to support the strategy planning team, under the leadership of Dr. Alex Gasasira, then WHO country representative to Liberia. Members of the Liberian legislature were invited to orientation sessions with the legal drafting team before the bill was submitted to them. The intention was to improve advocacy and promote information-sharing among lawmakers, whose constitutional mandates include law-making, oversight, and representation.

In December 2016, the bill to establish the NPHIL was passed by the Liberian Senate and the House of Representatives. It was signed into law by President Sirleaf on January 26, 2017, making this the date the NPHIL was officially established. The act established NPHIL as an autonomous government agency that would support activities of the minister of health. NPHIL would have oversight by a board of directors. The Ministry of Health and Social Welfare is represented on the board by the chief medical officer. The act amended a 1972 law to transfer the public health research function of the Ministry of Health to NPHIL and identified proposed funding sources for NPHIL, including budgetary allocation, fees for sale of research products, grants and donations, indirect costs on all grants, consulting and services fees, cooperative agreements, intellectual property, and establishment of an NPHIL Foundation.

There were several factors that favored the establishment of the NPHIL. There was immense support from the president of Liberia, the minister of health, a politically savvy deputy minister, and strategic technical partnerships with WHO, NIH, the CDC, and the International Association of National Public Health Institutes.

Many public health agencies around the world were founded after a health crisis. For example, Public Health Agency of Canada (PHAC)'s *Learning from SARS, Renewal of Public Health in Canada*, a report of the National Advisory Committee on SARS and Public Health, published in October 2003, and other Canadian and international reports recommended clear federal leadership on issues concerning public health.[12] The US CDC was founded to combat malaria;[13] Public Health England was a result of reorganization of the National Health Services in England for national protection of infectious diseases and substance misuse and abuse;[14] the Africa Centres for Disease Control and Prevention (Africa CDC) was established to support public health initiatives of member states and strengthen the capacity of their public health institutions to detect, prevent, control, and respond quickly and effectively to disease threats. Africa CDC was established in January 2016 and launched in January 2017, after the Ebola crisis in West Africa.[15]

NPHIL was established to strengthen public health surveillance, monitoring, and prevention of diseases with epidemic potential; bolster the country's response to outbreaks; augment existing infection prevention and control efforts; increase the capacity of existing laboratories; and build public health human resource capacity. NPHIL partners with the WHO, the CDC, the African Field Epidemiology Training Network, and the International Association of National Public Health Institutes.

Financing from the US government enabled construction of a new state-of-the-art reference laboratory and headquarters of the NPHIL in Monrovia. On October 5, 2017, President Ellen Johnson Sirleaf, US Ambassador Christian Elder, and Farid Zarif, special representative of the UN secretary-general, among other dignitaries, attended a groundbreaking for the NPHIL's construction at a site opposite the Ministry of Health at SKD Boulevard Junction in Congo Town, Monrovia.

NPHIL quickly became a center of excellence for better health outcomes for Liberians. The health care delivery system was restored in the nation's fifteen counties. Triages were built in most major hospitals and health centers. Water sanitation and hygiene services were restored; immunization services, malaria prevention and control, and HIV/AIDS and tuberculosis services also resumed. Community health workers and community health assistants were trained to provide and monitor basic health services to remote communities. The Liberia Institute for Biomedical Research (LIBR) facilities were revitalized with the capacity to test for over sixteen priority diseases, including Lassa fever, meningitis, measles, cholera, bloody diarrhea, influenza-like illnesses, meningococcal, and Ebola (which previously could not be tested in Liberia); COVID-19 was added to the list in 2020, after the onset of the COVID-19 pandemic.

In 2014, the Liberia-US Partnership for Research on Ebola Virus in Liberia (PREVAIL) was formed to conduct clinical research on Ebola therapeutics and vaccines. In February 2015, under the leadership of Dr. Anthony Fauci and Dr. H. Clifford Lane, PREVAIL launched a randomized placebo-controlled trial to assess the safety and efficacy of two experimental vaccines against Ebola: cAd3-EBOZ, developed by the NIAID, and Merck's RVSV-ZEBOV, developed with the Public Health Agency of Canada.[16] I was the Executive Committee chairman of

PREVAIL in Liberia. As chairman, I oversaw the political and technical role of the partnership and was responsible for leading the multimillion-dollar research enterprise, sponsored by NIAID. Because of these efforts, the world now has an efficacious Ebola vaccine that is currently being used in Ebola flare-ups in Liberia, Guinea, and the Democratic Republic of Congo.

In June 2015, I moved my family to the United States because our lives were threatened by Liberians who had lost family members to Ebola. Many who became ill and recovered with one malady or another, as well as others who felt that in my role as incident manager I could have done more to ease their pains, threatened our lives. They felt that I could have better controlled the situation and prevented further havoc in the country. They even expressed that they would deliberately infect me and my entire family. Consequently, my home and family were under the protection of armed police twenty-four hours a day. We were all afraid, so I decided to get them out of Liberia.

In October 2019, after twenty years of public service, I resigned my post as director general for extenuating circumstances and family reasons and joined my family in the United States.

In February 2020, I signed an employment agreement with the US Department of Health and Human Services (HHS) and National Institutes of Health (NIH) through an Intergovernmental Personnel Act (IPA). The IPA Mobility Program enables an exchange of skilled personnel between government and nongovernment institutions.[17] In my case, I was deployed to the Johns Hopkins Bloomberg School of Public Health, Department of International Health, with a rank of senior research associate. For me, Johns Hopkins was a familiar environment. I had maintained contact with faculty members, including Dr. David Peters, the chair of the Department of International Health, and Sara Bennett, director of the Health System Program. Dr. Peters participated in Liberia's Ebola response and, through the CDC, helped Liberia with its surveillance and data analysis. David and I coauthored articles on the epidemic that have been published in peer-reviewed journals and particular to crisis management: (1) "Financing Common Goods for Health: Core Government Functions in Health Emergency and Disaster Risk Management,"[18] and (2) "Leadership in Times of Crisis: The Example of Ebola Virus Disease in Liberia."[19]

Since the inception of the Global Health Security Index (GHSI) in 2016, I have been a member on the panel of experts. The index provides an assessment of global health security capabilities prepared by the Johns Hopkins Center for Health Security, the Nuclear Threat Initiative, and the Economist Intelligence Unit.[20] The twenty-one-member panel of international experts comprises public health experts, epidemiologists, scientists, academicians, legal scholars, the public and private sectors, and executive officers. In its assessment of 195 countries, the GHSI scored the United States number one in the world for readiness and preparedness. However, the haphazard US response to the COVID-19 pandemic was absolutely unbelievable to me! How could the United States, whose CDC travels the globe telling other countries how to manage epidemics and other public health incidents, lose control of this crisis? They were quite ineffective in doing exactly what they direct others to do: conduct an effective outbreak response with heightened surveillance, contact tracing, and infection prevention and control (IPC). They seemed ill prepared to contain the pandemic from the start.

On the political front, then president Donald J. Trump also seemed not to know what to do or who to consult and did not handle the initial COVID-19 crisis well at all. The public sense of confusion and uncertainty was palpable. Who could they trust? Who or what could they believe? The CDC, responsible for disease control and prevention, or President Trump and the political machinery? Unfortunately, neither could assure the American public that things were under control and the rapid escalation in infected cases and deaths in a matter of a few weeks didn't help matters either.

This reminded me of a similar situation in Liberia in July 2014, when the citizens felt that the government was mismanaging the Ebola response. People believed that the government was clueless about how to handle the epidemic. When the cases escalated and death toll exceeded 2,000 during July–September, the people did not hesitate to take to the streets expressing their fears and uncertainties. They demanded the resignation of the entire government, beginning with President Sirleaf stepping down. Opposition politicians had a field day, as they did in the United States with COVID-19, accusing the government of doing little or nothing to halt the outbreak. Politicians and citizens alike demanded that the government turn over the management of the response to the international community, as the public's conviction that the government did not know what to do intensified.

The similarity in initial outbreak response between Liberia (Ebola) and the United States (COVID-19) convinced me, as written in our "Leadership in Times of Crisis" article, that there is "no substitute for political leadership" in any outbreak and pandemic response.[19] It is obvious that governments must make concerted efforts to continuously monitor and evaluate their preparedness and response capabilities to disease outbreaks. In the United States, the COVID-19 pandemic explicitly demonstrated weaknesses in leadership to the initial public health response, same as what happened in Liberia with Ebola. In a broader sense, the pandemic showed the hollowness of the global health rhetoric of equity, the weaknesses of a health security–driven global health agenda, and the negative health impacts of power differentials on all fronts—globally, regionally, and locally.[21]

In his book *The End of Epidemics: The Looming Threat to Humanity and How to Stop It*, Jonathan D. Quick, MD,[22] mentioned the work that we did in Liberia during the Ebola epidemic response. In reference to President Ellen Johnson Sirleaf's leadership at that time, he indicated that, "when leaders learn deeply from their mistakes, they can also turn things around."[22] He noted that "President Sirleaf declared a national emergency and moved quickly to install a high-level pandemic response commander to lead the fight against the disease in Liberia." This she did after spending several months forming task forces and committees, trying to figure out what to do and how best to approach the national response, until mid-August, after 2,000 people had died and the public was calling for her entire government to step down. For a country with a population of a little over 4 million people at the time, losing 2,000 people was significant. Dr. Quick also described me as "a no-nonsense professional . . . obsessed with making things happen,"[22] and [he] "ran the organization from the top down, military style, as was appropriate during the emergency. There was one command center and one commander."[22] With this approach, we were able to end the Ebola outbreak in Liberia.

In response to the US COVID-19 crisis, I teamed up with other experts to develop the Johns Hopkins COVID-19 Contact Tracing Course. Initially we created the course for New York State, during the height of the pandemic. Before we began developing the course, I had several meetings, webinars, and presentations with state governors, their staff, state health departments, and secretaries of health about the importance of contact tracing. In the United States, contact tracing was practically nonexistent, meaning it was neither aggressive nor consistent—one of the key reasons for the widespread infection rates. This was surprising again, given the CDC's role in directing virtually every outbreak response internationally; here, in their own country, they seemed powerless to get a handle on the pandemic of the century. To those of us from other countries who experienced the CDC machinery in action, they appeared to have lost their way. I realized once more that they came to our countries to learn from us about effective outbreak response, just as we learned from them about their sophisticated techniques and methods. In responding to the West African Ebola epidemic, our three countries did better in containing the outbreak to prevent a massive global spread than the recognized experts of the great United States of America.

The three-hour online course was developed and launched to train an army of contact tracers. It was made available on Coursera, to anyone, at no cost, beginning May 11, 2020. Bloomberg Philanthropies funded the course development and free global access. By its one-year anniversary in 2021, the course had over 2.2 million viewers, including 1.2 million people who enrolled and received certificates of completion.[23] As of December 2022, 1.4 million people have received certificates of completion.[24] This COVID-19 contact tracing course teaches the basics of interviewing people diagnosed with the virus, identifying their close contacts who might have been exposed, and providing them guidance to self-quarantine for two weeks.[23]

"Even if you stop one or two new infections, you're preventing many new cases down the line," Johns Hopkins infectious disease epidemiologist Emily Gurley, the lead instructor of the course, said during a press briefing.[23] According to Joshua Sharfstein, a vice dean at the Bloomberg School of Public Health at Johns Hopkins, "The free six-hour course is open to anyone but taking and passing it will be a requirement for thousands of contact tracers being hired by the State of New York to fight the pandemic." Within hours of its May 11, 2020, release, more than 400 people had registered for the course.[23]

Health systems cannot function well if they are not resilient. The fragility of health systems has never been of greater "interest—or importance—than at this moment, in the aftermath of the worst Ebola virus epidemic" and COVID-19 pandemic to date.[25] Health system resilience can be defined as the "capacity of health actors, institutions, and populations to prepare for and effectively respond to crises; maintain core functions when a crisis hits; and, informed by lessons learned during the crisis, reorganize if conditions require it."[25] Health systems are resilient if they "protect human life and produce good health outcomes for all during a crisis and in its aftermath. Resilient health systems can also deliver everyday benefits and positive health outcomes. This double benefit—improved performance in both bad times and good—is what has been called "the resilience dividend."[25]

The takeaway message here, as we have learned in low- and middle-income settings, is that leading a national crisis response carries a tremendous responsibility. Everyone looks to you for a rapid solution to end the crisis. In my case, the responsibility was even greater, not just for the government.[26] My family also felt the tremendous weight of my leadership as incident manager and the magnitude of the threats on our lives. The intensity of their fear that I might be directly exposed to

EVD and bring it home, risking infecting everyone in our household,[26] forced me to consider separating myself from my young children and my beloved wife. Painfully, I made the tough decision to send them to the United States for safekeeping, so to speak. It was worrisome yet, deep in my soul, I knew that I had to remain in Liberia to undertake the task for which I had been preparing all my life—from the moment of my birth, when my father had the vision of me becoming a leader for my country.

CHAPTER 10

Reflections

As we reflect on the dreams we had, the great things we imagined for ourselves and our children—the joys, excitement, career highs and lows, frustrations, and disappointments along the way—we recognize that the role we played in the Ebola response in Liberia was one of the most rewarding and demanding experiences of our lives. It was a pivotal moment, a definite career high, something we dreamed of though not envisioned it in quite the manner it manifested. Yet, it was one for which we had been preparing for a very long time. As Ellen Johnson Sirleaf said in delivering her commencement speech to Harvard University's graduating class of 2011, "The size of your dreams must always exceed your current capacity to achieve them. If your dreams do not scare you, they are not big enough. If you start off with a small dream, you may not have much left when it is fulfilled because along the way, life will task your dreams and make demands on you."[1]

The initial efforts by the government of Liberia were fragmented. There were three task forces: the National Ebola Task Force, chaired by President Sirleaf, the MOHSW task force led by then minister of health Walter Gwenigale (deceased 2022), and the logistics task force, jointly led by Mary Broh, director general of the General Services Agency, and

Dorbor Jallah, manager of the Ebola Trust Fund. Each task force functioned independently, with offices in different locations in Monrovia. Consequently, coordination of response activities was disjointed and plagued by ineffectiveness as infection rates soared, with close to 2,000 lives lost between July and September 2014. The death of so many Liberians in such a short time span was the catalyst that convinced President Sirleaf to act more decisively by disbanding the three task forces and making the necessary change from uncoordinated, independently led task forces, to a one command and control IMS system. How did she arrive at that point? In his blog, Rony Zagursky asked the question, "Do leaders only hear what they want to hear, or do they listen to what they need to hear?"[2] Was the president ever told that the change was essential? If so, was she only hearing what she wanted to hear, until the situation became so grave that she was forced to listen and then heard what she needed to hear? David Fubini addresses leadership issues in his book *Hidden Truths: What Leaders Need to Hear But Are Rarely Told*.[3] He writes, "When leaders know the right time to leave, their companies benefit, and . . . the leaders themselves are also beneficiaries. They depart with their legacy intact and their reputations secured. . . . It might seem that smart and savvy leaders would recognize that timing is everything. Unfortunately, even the brightest can only see what they want to see."[3] Making the change from the MOHSW Task Force to the IMS structure was a decisive factor in President Sirleaf's leadership, when she began to regard the Ebola virus disease as a threat to the nation's "economic, political and social fabric" and when she made the response a definite priority for multiple branches of her government. Thereafter, her swift and sometimes tough decisions, frequent public pronouncements, and presence at outbreak sites were demonstrative of this leadership.

The lessons we learned about crisis leadership were profound. There are several key principles that have practical relevance, as outlined in my article, "Leadership in Times of Crisis: A Personal Reflection from the Hot Seat of the Ebola Epidemic Response in Liberia": "There is no substitute for political leadership," "To lead effectively, there must be a supporting cast," "Governments must take ownership of their response," "It is critical that systems and structures be put in place early," and "The relationship with international partners must be managed well if it is to work."[4]

President Sirleaf's decisive leadership at that time demonstrated that, indeed, there is no substitute for political leadership. Her support to the IMS team was unwavering, and her government stepped up, took ownership of their response, and managed the national crisis as a political priority, while embracing the cultural and political context of the country. With the backing of the political apparatus, the IMS strategy was effective. Teamwork was fundamental to our success, with our technical teams serving as the supporting cast. We each had a specific role to play.[4] We knew undoubtedly that our lives were on the line and we had more to lose than anyone else—especially so, when in October 2014 the UN estimated that foreign nationals participating in the response would constitute only 2%. Therefore, we Liberians had to take charge of saving our own lives.[5]

Navigating our way in dealing with the influx of the multitude of foreign entities was taxing, because we didn't have the requisite systems and infrastructure to accommodate all these people. Navigating the multiplicity of relationships and partnerships with these foreign entities, in what became a multinational and multidisciplinary response, had its complexities and had to be handled delicately, because they came with the package of expertise, and financial and logistical assistance. For these reasons, we opened our doors wide, allowing them to have full access, participating in decision-making and consensus, often without question. Yet, we expected them to understand the political context and be respectful of the government's strategic direction. Sometimes they were not. We expected them to respect the culture and tradition of the people they came to assist. Sometimes they did not. We expected them to be accountable with regard to resource allocation. Sometimes they were not forthcoming. We also expected them to be honest in sharing their specific program design and activity implementation plans or strategies. Some entities were not. In several instances, we discovered that some came with their own interests and agendas—they were independently soliciting funds and other resources in the name of Liberia, when all along the government was never consulted and therefore was completely unaware. This sort of solicitation was in the sole interest of the entity soliciting, for their own benefit, with the singular intention of enriching themselves. Many refused to share the details with us once the government became aware of their inappropriate, unauthorized solicitation. Ebola became fair game, a get-rich-quick scheme; unfortunately, many newly established entities managed to infiltrate the system and reaped a fortune at our expense. It became imperative to constantly remind partners and friends alike of our slogan: *One Plan, One Strategy, One Response.* Further on, collaborative engagement—conferring jointly on solving problems—yielded better results and the government could then more readily request or delegate responsibility to an agency in instances where the national team's technical capacity in specific areas was minimal or nonexistent. At best, this meant integrating national and foreign teams to work as a unit, on one specified thematic strategy.

Our skills and extraordinary leadership were only recognized by our foreign partners when the situation began to improve. At that point, it became obvious to us that the so-called foreign experts didn't know any more about managing Ebola than we did. Many of them came to gain experience to claim their expertise, writing and publishing papers at our expense. We even discovered that although we were doing the bulk of the work—98% in reality—they were writing papers without one mention of our names, until my able advisor, Dr. Mardia Stone—a WHO consultant seconded to my office as senior and technical advisor—alerted me to what was occurring. She informed me that we too—our core team of Liberian professionals—were becoming Ebola experts and that we had to control the outflow of papers written on our response. She advised that we needed our names on these papers to truly be considered experts in the field and if we did not, the academic and research worlds would never consider us as such. With her guidance, we took the position that every paper written on Liberia's Ebola response by participating international partners and agencies required our participation in the formation of ideas, drafting, and editing. Furthermore, each draft of a scientific paper had to be presented for my approval.

We were stunned by the strong resistance posed by leaders of some agencies regarding getting our names included on these papers in the first place, and then, who would be first, second, or third author on any given paper. We argued our position that Liberians should be given first, second, third, and senior authorship on most, though not all, papers—and we definitely had to insist on it. That is how Liberian members of the IMS core team were included as coauthors on multiple scientific writings on Liberia's Ebola response. We were of the conviction that we too should benefit from our labor and should not have to struggle or fight to get our names on the papers written about the hard work we did collectively, as Liberians. It was then that the politics, deception, and greed in public health and intellectual property of research papers became very clear to us. From that point onward, we committed ourselves to being more self-reliant, advocating for our cause.

In many ways, for Liberians, Ebola was a blessing in disguise. We learned that humility was an essential element in working with diverse groups of people. By being humble, we could accomplish much more. Prior to Ebola, many of us who worked in the Ministry of Health and Social Welfare had limited professional exposure to, or significant interactions with, foreign partners. We interacted mainly among ourselves and with very few foreign experts. We did not socialize with them either. The epidemic had many complexities. It brought nationals and foreigners together in professional relationships, giving us the opportunity to work side-by-side. I realized then that when one is innately a leader, opportunities for leadership emerge. Case in point is my appointment as incident manager, based on my demonstrated leadership and my bosses' and President Sirleaf's observance of my ability to lead. I didn't comprehend it at first, until I realized that this monumental Ebola crisis presented a tremendous opportunity for me to truly become a recognized leader. There will be other major public health events in time. Today, however, the experience of the West African

Ebola outbreak is reshaping the future of public health for Liberia and the world at large.

Elections in the Midst of An Epidemic

Just as COVID-19 affected electoral voting in the United States in November 2020, Liberia's Senatorial elections scheduled for December 20, 2014, were also affected by Ebola. Voter turnout was expected to be high in the United States, even after a long period of restrictions by the government, which kept public gatherings at a minimum; the same was expected in Liberia, where an absentee or mail-in ballot system does not exist. As in the United States, politicians in Liberia contesting reelection, with both the fear of losing and fearing for overall safety of themselves and voters, wanted the elections canceled. On the flip side of the coin, politicians in their very first electoral race, hoping to unseat incumbent senators, demanded that elections be held as scheduled. The IMS team assured the government that new strategies and logistics would be developed in concert with the National Elections Commission (NEC) to ensure that elections were safe. A series of new protocols, regulations, additional staffing, and equipment—hand-washing stations and thermometers—were instituted at polling stations across the country. Extra hand sanitizers were also available. There were procedures to obtain telephone numbers of each voter, in case contact tracing became necessary. Despite extremely challenging logistics, we were able to convince NEC, political leaders, and the President's Advisory Committee on Ebola (PACE) that it was safe to conduct the elections, thereby preventing political standoff and instability in the nation.

Services and Schools

In Liberia, social services and school systems were critically impacted by Ebola, as has been the case with the COVID-19 pandemic in the United States. Schools were closed nationwide due to fears of EVD exposure and potential widespread transmission in schools. Health officials recommended against complete school closure. They argued that training teachers on new school health safety protocols, educating students on these safety procedures, proper hand-washing techniques, social distancing, and intensifying school health safety monitoring activities were better disease preventive measures. Therefore, they supported school reopening, based on active implementation of these preventive measures nationally. They also made the case that young students' education and social development skills would be stalled if they were isolated from their peers for prolonged periods. Because Ebola is a hemorrhagic disease, transmitted mainly by direct physical contact to an infected person or infected corpse—touching or exposure to infected body fluids—and not a respiratory illness like COVID-19, mask wearing was not necessary. School closure also halted related economic activities, creating financial hardship for many merchants. Health officials suggested parents be encouraged to share responsibility in educating their children to protect themselves from EVD. There were also budgetary implications for procurement of supplies and equipment—soap, thermometers, tents and so on. The IMS facilitated all of these measures.

Getting the Community Involved

Social mobilization is defined as "the primary step of community development for recovery from conflicts and disasters. It allows people to think and understand their situation and to organize and initiate action for their recovery with their own initiative and creativity."[1] In our situation, social mobilization, community engagement, and awareness were fundamental to the success of the Ebola epidemic response. We used a bottom to top, all-societal approach, by actively engaging traditional and religious leaders (Muslims and Christians), as well as traditional healers, to clearly understand traditional behavior and norms related to rituals for the dead. We needed to understand in order to discourage them from directly handling infected corpses (bathing the dead and exposing the living to their infected bodily fluids and bath-water). It was interesting to learn that these traditionalists never once considered the possibility of transmitting disease through practices that are common to them yet are unconventional and unacceptable to others. They were also stubborn in their refusal to comply with government directives until they witnessed the death of whole households and family members daily. Then in fear, they heard our plea and complied.

COVID-19 Response—Liberia

Liberia's first COVID-19 case was recorded and confirmed on March 16, 2020.[6] The Ministry of Health reported that a forty-six-year-old male Liberian national traveled to Switzerland on official duty on March 9, 2020, and returned home on March 13, 2020, via SN Brussels Airlines, flight 241. According to the situation report, on March 14, the patient reported onset of symptoms (fever and unproductive cough) to authorities. On March 15, he sought over-the-counter medication from Lucky Pharmacy, in Monrovia; at about 10:43 a.m., the patient reported to the National Public Health Institute of Liberia (NPHIL), where a laboratory sample was collected and sent to the National Reference Laboratory (NRL) for testing. On March 16, 2020, at about 3:00 a.m., NRL confirmed the patient's lab specimen was positive for COVID-19 (a twenty-four-hour turnaround time), making this the index case for COVID-19 in Liberia. This is a remarkable improvement in collection, testing, and reporting time, compared to the early days of the Ebola outbreak (March–August 2014), when it took several weeks to get results, even a month, whether positive or negative. Testing capacity at that time in the country was nonexistent. Ebola samples were transported to Médecins Sans Frontières (MSF; also known as Doctors Without Borders) facilities in Guinea and then to Lyon, France, for testing. Transporting samples from remote locations was very difficult due to logistics (vehicles, transport media).[7]

The experience from the Ebola epidemic prepared Liberia, in many ways, for any future epidemic or pandemic—hence, its effective response to the COVID-19 pandemic. For example, when Ebola first emerged in West Africa, leaders scrambled to design and implement a system that could mount an effective response. Ebola forced the government of Liberia to honestly assess its own frail health infrastructure in a multiplicity of ways. Under immense pressure, establishing an incident management system and response structures in all counties, and investing in a National Reference Laboratory and regional reference laboratories in five other counties, resulted in reliable, rapid testing capacities. This is what we saw when the first COVID-19 case was diagnosed and confirmed in March 2020. An aggressive approach to contact tracing, educating, and engaging the community in the process made it easier for us to find Ebola-infected community members who were obviously ill, dying, or in hiding. Communicating the nature and risks of Ebola in simple terms, in colloquial or "simple English" as they say in Liberia, in vernacular, through graphic poster illustrations, and drama, in some instances, led the community to better understand the risks to which they were exposed, fostering a more resilient community. Ultimately, taking steps to enact a law establishing the NPHIL—mandated as the umbrella of disease surveillance, prevention, and control of public health risks, epidemic preparedness, and response—consolidated all of those successful strategic mechanisms under one roof. Together, all these enhanced the COVID-19 response in 2020. Consequently, Liberia had very low caseloads and minimal case fatalities, reporting 6,795 cases and 248 deaths from March 2020 to December 2021, twenty-one months into the COVID-19 pandemic, compared to 11,000 cases and over 4,803 deaths in twenty-four months of the Ebola epidemic. However, it is important to note here that the epidemiology of the two diseases is not the same, even though many strategies from the Ebola response are applicable to the COVID-19 response. In mounting a response this time around, the Liberian team was proactive, compared to being reactive, when Ebola struck. They initiated early testing, aggressive contact tracing, rapid isolation of patients, and immediate points-of-entry (POE) screening at airports, seaports, and across borders. Community engagement and social mobilization was initiated, and health care workers were trained and practiced infection prevention control (IPC) and treatment techniques. Personal protective equipment (PPEs) was readily available and utilized. Yet, despite the progress made, Liberia remains vulnerable, to a degree, in future epidemic preparedness and response due to continuing health system weaknesses.

COVID-19 Response—United States

By all accounts, numerous errors were made in the United States' initial COVID-19 response, which became more fragmented as infection and death rates skyrocketed. The COVID-19 Task Force seemed not to have a clear incident manager nor a clear command-and-control incident management system (IMS) in place. The same occurred in Liberia during the early stages of Ebola. There were mixed messages coming from various US government (USG) sources, while Vice President Mike Pence was supposedly the lead or incident manager. Messages regarding mask wearing were inconsistent. Contact tracing apparently was not emphasized nor conducted routinely. In short, there was no decisive leadership in the midst of the US pandemic response.

The CDC, which played a leading role as our partner in the Ebola response, even recommending the set up for an incident management system, seemed to be paralyzed—or so it appeared to us Africans. They were busy telling us what to do and how to manage our response, yet when the time came to implement all that "expert advice" they constantly give to other countries, they failed at doing the same for their own country. What happened here? As Africans, we felt that CDC had no voice in its country's COVD-19 response. As the public health agency of the US government, the CDC should have been the incident manager and managed the federal government response. At least, based on experience, that would have been their message to us.

When President Trump took the lead at daily briefings, it became a top-down, highly political approach, which was disruptive. He assumed the role of incident manager. That also was the experience in Liberia, until the escalating cases and death rates redirected the thinking of our president and her government and, upon the advice of the US CDC (yes, they did advise), to a clear command-and-control incident management system (IMS) with a designated incident manager. We adopted a bottom to top, all-societal approach by actively engaging the community and traditional and religious leaders. In our situation, contact tracing, social mobilization, community engagement, and awareness were fundamental to the success of the Ebola epidemic response.

A vast landscape (3.797 million square miles) and a much larger population (over 350 million people) posed difficulties for US officials in contact tracing; in contrast, Liberia's 4.5 million people reside in 43,000 square miles, making door-to-door contact tracing possible. However, in a society as technologically sophisticated as the United States, a contact tracing mechanism could have been implemented as the CDC did for those of us entering US airports during the Ebola epidemic from West Africa. We were isolated in designated screening rooms at the airport, especially the John F. Kennedy International Airport in New York, where most flights from West Africa arrived. Once in the isolated room, our temperatures were taken, then we were questioned about everything we did (seemed like one's whole life) before getting on that flight to JFK. Once cleared, each person was given a phone—a tracker of sorts—to call in and report daily temperature checks, signs, and symptoms, if any, to a CDC-designated person for twenty-one days, the Ebola incubation period. Liberians called it the Ebola tracking phone.

Key lessons we learned that were missing in the US COVID-19 response is that political leadership cannot be substituted in responding to public health crisis, but "to lead effectively, there must be a supporting cast."[4] Governments must take ownership of their response, and "it is critical that systems and structures be put in place early."[4] With the unwavering support of our president, the IMS strategy was effective. We operated as a team, a fundamental element to our success, with each technical team playing a specific role.[4] Our slogan—*One Plan, One Strategy, One Response*—conveyed the government's position that everyone had to be on the same page. It worked! And so, this, in addition to the strategies we outlined earlier, constitutes our approach to all future epidemics.

In Recognition of African Scientists

In further reflection, we recall the story of the Congolese epidemiologist Dr. Jean-Jacques Muyembe, who first discovered "a mysterious disease in central Congo in 1976"[8] and collected and sent viral samples to Belgium for analysis.[8] The analysis was done by Belgian doctors, including Dr. Peter Piot, who is now well recognized as the "discoverer" of Ebola, along with Dr. Guido van der Groen.[9,10] Despite receiving the viral samples from Dr. Muyembe, neither of the two scientists ever mentioned his name or credited him as the original discoverer of the Ebola virus. They took all the credit and built their careers on it as Western colonialist always did, and as is still being done today, regardless of the professional capabilities of African scientists across the continent. That's why we choose to recognize Dr. Jean-Jacques Muyembe as a blessing to Liberia. He came to Liberia with his team of five other Congolese scientists and medics when we were lost. Their arrival was timely. He helped us make sense of Ebola and made us realize that we, Liberians, had the capacity to do the job and, with the proper guidance, we could succeed in curbing Ebola. By willingly sharing his knowledge, experience, and expertise with us, he actually helped us change the dynamics of the lethal disease and helped us turn things around in beating Ebola out of Liberia. What was most obvious to us is that African scientists who came to Liberia had more knowledge, experience, and better skills in dealing with Ebola than the non-Africans who came from across the globe to assist us. For that reason, we give credit and express our sincere gratitude to our fellow Africans who came to our aid, in various capacities—some of whom, for so long, have worked in the shadows of others, until now. They stepped up to the plate and helped us save our country from annihilation by Ebola, the virus that broke every rule once it hit West Africa.

Conclusion

Despite the horrific experiences we had as a nation during the epidemic, Liberians still had hope. They continued to live their lives, even with the restrictions on common human interactions—no touching, no hugging, no kissing, no hand shaking, no gathering when a loved one died, no funerals. The horror of cremation, so foreign to the society, induced more fear that people would burn in hell. Yet there was hope. And so, when a group of Liberians and expatriates organized the third Monrovia Marathon, announcing in mid-July that Sunday, November 8, 2015, would be "A New Beginning,"[11] the theme of the event, people saw a reason to participate and celebrate life. The first Monrovia Marathon launched in 2011 and the second in 2013. There was no race in 2014 due to Ebola. This was a clear indication that this marathon, the first regional, multinational sporting event post-Ebola, would bring

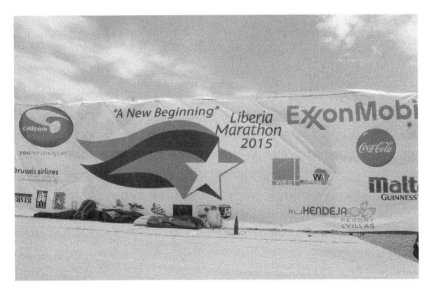

Monrovia Marathon banner

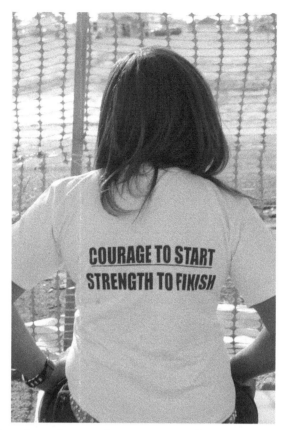

Courage to Start, Strength to Finish, Monrovia Marathon

people together once again, not just from within the boundaries of Liberia. They would come from as far away as Kenya, Senegal, and our Mano River Union neighbors, Sierra Leone and Guinea, with whom we also shared the classification of being the three most affected countries in the West African Ebola outbreak. There were 1,500 registered racers,[12] including those in wheelchairs and other handicapped racers. Runners from Sierra Leone won first and second place. A Liberian was third. There were all kinds of fashionable onlookers. Being in that space was exhilarating. It was truly a "new beginning," a fresh start, standing up against Ebola—and we won.

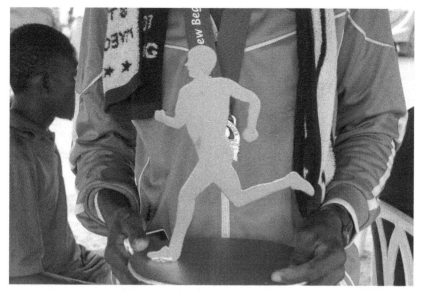

Going for the gold, Monrovia Marathon

In the words of the Liberian National Anthem, "In union strong, success assured, we will over all prevail, we will over all prevail, we will over all prevail. With hearts and hands our country's soil defending, we meet the foe, with valor unpretending. Long live Liberia."[13] We defended our country against the foe, and we prevailed when we succeeded in driving Ebola out of Liberia. Had we not moved swiftly to curb the disease, the Ebola epidemic could have become a disastrous pandemic. We put our lives on the line to save our country, and in so doing we saved the world.

ACRONYMS AND ABBREVIATIONS

ACDC	Africa Centres for Disease Control and Prevention
ACT	artemisinin-based combination therapy
ADRA	Adventist Development and Relief Agency
AFT	Agenda for Transformation
AIDS	acquired immunodeficiency syndrome
ASEOWA	African Union Support to Ebola in West Africa
AU	African Union
CBI	community-based initiative
CBRN	chemical, biological, radiological, or nuclear
CCC	community care center
CDC	US Centers for Disease Control and Prevention
CEBS	community event-based surveillance
CHA	community household approach
CHAP	Community Health Assistance Program
CHO	county health officer
CHT	county health team
CHV	community health volunteer
CHW	community health worker
CIA	US Central Intelligence Agency
CMO	chief medical officer
DAF	Dutch Truck Manufacturing
DART	Disaster Assistance Response Team (USAID)
DBM	Dead Body Management
DFID	Department for International Development (UK)
DG	director general
DHHS	Department of Health and Human Services (US)
DOD	US Department of Defense
DPD	Disease Prevention Division (part of MOHSW)
DRC	Democratic Republic of the Congo
DTRA	Defense Threat Reduction Agency

ECA	Economic Commission for Africa
ECAP	Ebola Community Action Platform
ECHO	European Commission's Humanitarian Aid and Civil Protection Department
ECOWAS	Economic Community of West African States
EERP	Ebola Emergency Response Project
EERP–AF	Emergency Ebola Response Project–Additional Financing
ELBC	Liberian Broadcasting System
ELISA	enzyme linked immunosorbent assay
ELWA	Eternal Love Winning Africa (entity running ELWA Hospital)
EOC	Emergency Operations Center
EPA	Environmental Protection Agency
EPI	Expanded Programme on Immunization
EPR	Epidemic Preparedness and Response
EPRP	Emergency Preparedness and Response Plan
ETU	Ebola treatment unit
EU	European Union
EVD	Ebola virus disease
EWARN	Early Warning, Alert and Response Network
FDA	US Food and Drug Administration
FEMA	Federal Emergency Management Agency (US)
FLB	forward logistics base
GDP	gross domestic product
GHSA	Global Health Security Agenda
GHSI	Global Health Security Index
HIV	human immunodeficiency virus
HMIS	Health Management Information System and Research
HSCC	Health Sector Coordination Committee
IANPHI	International Association of National Public Health Institutes
ICT	information and communication technology
IDA	International Development Association
IDSR	Integrated Disease Surveillance and Response
IFRC	International Federation of Red Cross
IHR	International Health Regulations
IMS	incident management system
IPC	infection prevention and control
IREX	International Research & Exchanges Board
JEE	Joint External Evaluation
KAP	knowledge, attitudes, and practices

LIBR	Liberia Institute for Biomedical Research
LISGIS	Liberia Institute for Statistics and Geo-Information Services
LMDC	Liberia Medical and Dental Council
LPC	Liberian Peace Council
MICAT	Ministry of Information, Cultural Affairs, and Tourism
MLB	main logistics base
MOFDP	Ministry of Finance and Development Planning
MOH	Ministry of Health
MOHSW	Ministry of Health and Social Welfare
MSF	Médecins Sans Frontières / Doctors Without Borders
MSU	mobile storage unit
MT	metric ton
NACP	National AIDS Control Program
NEC	National Elections Commission
NGOs	nongovernmental organizations
NIAID	National Institute of Allergy and Infectious Diseases
NIH	National Institutes of Health (US)
NMCP	National Malaria Control Program
NPHIL	National Public Health Institute of Liberia
NPR	National Public Radio
NRL	National Reference Laboratory
NTBCP	National Tuberculosis Control Program
OAU	Organization of African Unity
OFDA	Office of Foreign Disaster Assistance (USAID)
OPD	outpatient department
OUA	Operation United Assistance (US)
PACE	Presidential Advisory Council on Ebola
PAL	Progressive Alliance of Liberia
PCR	polymerase chain reaction
PHEIC	public health emergency of international concern
PI	principal investigator
PMI	President's Malaria Initiative (US)
POE	ports of entry
PPE	personal protective equipment
PRC	People's Redemption Council
PREVAIL	Partnership for Research on Ebola Virus in Liberia
PSC	Peace and Security Council
PSI	Population Services International
RED	reach every district

REDISSE	Regional Disease Surveillance System Enhancement
RIA	Roberts International Airport / Robertsfield
RITE	rapid isolation and treatment of Ebola
RMT	Response Management Team
RRL	Regional Reference Laboratory
RRT	Rapid Response Teams
SIM	Serving in Mission (a Christian organization)
SITTU	Severe Infection Temporary Treatment Unit
SKD	Samuel Kanyon Doe Sports Complex
SOE	state-owned enterprise
SOP	standard operating procedure
TOT	training of trainers
UDHR	Universal Declaration of Human Rights
UL	University of Liberia
UNAIDS	United Nations Programme on HIV/AIDS
UNDP	United Nations Development Programme
UNFPA	United Nations Population Fund
UNHCR	United Nations High Commission on Refugees
UNICEF	United Nations International Children's Emergency Fund
UNMEER	United Nations Mission for Ebola Emergency Response
UNOPS	United Nations Office of Project Services
USACE	US Army Corps of Engineers
USAID	United States Agency for International Development
USPHS	US Public Health Services
USSR	Union of Soviet Socialist Republics
VOTT	Voice of Tabou 11
WAHO	West African Health Organization
WASH	water, sanitation, and hygiene
WFP	World Food Programme
WHO	World Health Organization

INTRODUCTION

1. Sirleaf EJ. Statement by her excellency President Johnson Sirleaf on the update of the Ebola crisis. September 17, 2014. https://www.emansion.gov.lr/doc /Nation_Address-17092014.pdf

2. Begley S. Ebola cases could reach 550,000 to 1.4 mln by late Jan—CDC. Reuters. https://www.reuters.com/article/ozatp-us-health-ebola-cdc-idAFKCN0HI1UR20140923. Published September 23, 2014.

CHAPTER 1: Ebola Hits Liberia

1. Wikipedia contributors. West African Ebola virus epidemic. Wikipedia, The Free Encyclopedia. https://en.m.wikipedia.org/wiki/West_African_Ebola_virus _epidemic. March 15, 2019.

2. Meltzer MI, Atkins YC, Santibanez S, et al. Estimating the future number of cases in the Ebola epidemic—Liberia and Sierra Leone, 2014–2015. *CDC Morbidity and Mortality Weekly Report*. 2014;63(03):1–14. https://www.cdc.gov/mmwr/preview /mmwrhtml/su63e0923a1.htm

3. Worland J. WHO: New Ebola cases could hit 10,000 per week. *Time*. http://time .com/3505982/ebola-new-cases-world-health-organization. Published October 14, 2014.

4. Yan H, Smith E. Ebola: Patient zero was a toddler in Guinea. *CNN*. http:// edition.cnn.com/2014/10/28/health/ebola-patient-zero/index.html. Published January 21, 2015.

5. Baize S, Pannetier D, Oestereich L, et al. Emergence of Zaire Ebola virus disease in Guinea—preliminary report. *N Eng J Med*. 2014;371(15):1418–1425. https://doi.org/10.1056/NEJMoa1404505

6. Stylianou N. How world's worst Ebola outbreak began with one boy's death. BBC News. https://www.bbc.com/news/world-africa-30199004. Published November 27, 2014.

7. Liberia: A country—and its capital—are overwhelmed with Ebola cases. World Health Organization website. https://www.medbox.org/pdf/5e148832db60a2044 c2d3ab0. Published January 2015.

8. International Health Regulations. World Health Organization website. https://www.emro.who.int/health-topics/international-health-regulations/index .html. December 19, 2019.

9. What are the International Health Regulations and emergency committees? Q&A. World Health Organization website. December 19, 2019. https://www.who.int /news-room/questions-and-answers/item/emergencies-international-health -regulations-and-emergency-committees

10. Youde J. Biopolitical surveillance in the international arena. *In: Biopolitical Surveillance and Public Health in International Politics*. Palgrave Macmillan; 2010: 147–175. https://doi.org/10.1057/9780230104785_2

11. Kohl KS, Arthur RR, O'Connor R, Fernandez J. Assessment of public health events through international regulations, United States, 2007–2011. *Emerg Infect Dis.* 2012;18(7):1047–1053. https://doi.org/10.3201/eid1807.120231. PMID 22709566.

12. What is Ebola virus disease? US Centers for Disease Control and Prevention website. https://www.cdc.gov/vhf/ebola/about.html. Updated April 27, 2021.

13. Nyenswah TG, Kateh F, Bawo L, et al. Ebola and its control in Liberia, 2014–2015. *Emerg Infect Dis.* 2016;22(2):169–77. https://doi.org/10.3201/eid2202.151456

14. Ebola virus disease. US Centers for Disease Control and Prevention website. https://www.cdc.gov/vhf/ebola. Last modified May 15, 2018.

15. Coltart CE, Lindsey B, Ghinai I, Johnson AM, Heymann DL. The Ebola outbreak, 2013–2016: Old lessons for new epidemics. *Philos Trans Royal Soc Lond B Biol Sci.* 2017;372(1721):20160297. https://doi.org/10.1098/rstb.2016.0297

16. Ebola virus disease distribution map: Cases of Ebola virus disease in Africa since 1976. Centers for Disease Control and Prevention website. https://www.cdc.gov /vhf/ebola/history/distribution-map.html

17. Ebola virus disease factsheet. World Health Organization website. https:// www.who.int/news-room/fact-sheets/detail/ebola-virus-disease. Accessed November 2021.

18. Ebola (Ebola virus disease): Signs and symptoms. US Centers for Disease Control and Prevention website. https://www.cdc.gov/vhf/ebola/symptoms/index.html

19. Survivors. US Centers for Disease Control and Prevention website. https:// www.cdc.gov/vhf/ebola/treatment/survivors.html. Last updated November 5, 2019.

20. Key events in the WHO response to the Ebola outbreak. World Health Organization website. https://www.who.int/news-room/spotlight/one-year-into-the -ebola-epidemic/key-events-in-the-who-response-to-the-ebola-outbreak. Published January 2015.

21. Senga M, Pringle K, Ramsay A, et al. Factors underlying Ebola virus infection among health workers, Kenema, Sierra Leone, 2014–2015. *Clin Infect Dis.* 2016;63(4):454–459. https://doi.org/10.1093/cid/ciw327

22. United Nations Development Programme, Human Development Report 2020, http://hdr.undp.org/en/countries/profiles/LBR

23. Liberia GDP per capita. Trading Economics website. https://tradingeconomics .com/liberia/gdp-per-capita

24. Liberia Institute of Statistics and Geo-Information Service (LISGIS), Ministry of Health [Liberia], and ICF. *Liberia Demographic and Health Survey 2019–2020.* https://www.dhsprogram.com/pubs/pdf/FR362/FR362.pdf

25. Rubenstein L. *Perilous Medicine: The Struggle to Protect Health Care from Violence*. Columbia University Press; 2021: 220.

26. Witt JF. Two conceptions of suffering in war. In: Sarat A, ed. *Knowing the Suffering of Others: Legal Perspectives on Pain and its Meaning*. University of Alabama Press; 2014.

27. World Health Assembly, Resolution 46.39, Sanitary and Medical Services in Times of Armed Conflict, WHA46.39 (May 14, 1993). https://apps.who.int/iris/handle/10665/176491

28. Arwady MA, Bawo L, Hunter JC, et al. Evolution of Ebola virus disease from exotic infection to global health priority, Liberia, mid-2014. *Emerg Infect Dis.* 2015;21(4):578–584.

29. World Health Organization's Global Health Workforce Statistics: Physicians (Per 1,000 People). World Bank website. http://data.worldbank.org/indicator/. Accessed May 19, 2017.

30. Ministry of Health. *Investment Plan for Building a Resilient Health System: 2015–2021*. May 12, 2015. https://au.int/web/sites/default/files/newsevents/workingdocuments/27027-wd-liberia-_investment_plan_for_building_a_resilient_health_system.pdf

31. MSF Report. The failures of the international outbreak response. https://www.msf.org/ebola-failures-international-outbreak-response

CHAPTER 2: Born for Such a Time

1. Jackson SP. *Rich Land Poor Country: The "Paradox of Poverty" in Liberia*. Samuel P. Jackson; 2019: 315–375.

2. Hahn N. US covert and overt operations in Liberia, 1970s to 2003. *ASPJ Africa & Francophonie*. Third Quarter 2014:20. https://www.airuniversity.af.edu/Portals/10/ASPJ_French/journals_E/Volume-05_Issue-3/Hahn_e.pdf

3. Tolbert WR Jr. President Tolbert's speech at Nkrumah Symposium, May 13, 1972. In: *Presidential Papers, Documents, Diary, and Records of Activities of the Chief Executive, First Year of the Administration of President William R. Tolbert Jr., 23 July 1971–31 July 1972*, ed. Executive Mansion (Monrovia), 511.

4. Organization of African Unity, *Monrovia Declaration of Commitment of the Heads of State and Government, of the Organization of African Unity on Guidelines and Measures for National and Collective Self-Reliance in Social and Economic Development for the Establishment of a New International Economic Order*, in *AHG/ST. 3 (XVI)*, rev.1, ed. Organization of African Unity (Monrovia: African Union, 1979), 5, point 6.

5. Arrighi G. The African crisis: World systemic and regional aspects. *New Left Review*. May & June 2002;15:5–36. https://newleftreview.org/issues/ii15/articles/giovanni-arrighi-the-african-crisis.pdf

6. Accelerated development in Sub-Saharan Africa: An agenda for action. World Bank. https://documents.worldbank.org/en/publication/documents-reports/documentdetail/702471468768312009/accelerated-development-in-sub-saharan-africa-an-agenda-for-action. Published January 1, 1981.

7. Nyenswah T. Interview with Wesley M. Johnson, Liberian ambassador to the UK. December 6, 2010. Mr. Johnson was vice chairman, INTG, 2003–2006; vice chairman, People's Progressive Party (PPP), 1978–1990, and subsequently chairman.

CHAPTER 3: Unsafe Rituals, Burial Practices, and International Spread

1. Liberia: A country—and its capital—are overwhelmed with Ebola cases. World Health Organization. One Year Report on Ebola, January 2015. https://www.who.int /news-room/spotlight/one-year-into-the-ebola-epidemic/liberia-a-country-and-its -capital-are-overwhelmed-with-ebola-cases. Retrieved November 7, 2021.

2. Wikipedia contributors. First Consultant Hospital. Wikipedia, The Free Encyclopedia. July 20, 2022, 16:33 UTC. https://en.wikipedia.org/w/index.php?title =First_Consultant_Hospital&oldid=1099409427

3. Wikipedia contributors. Patrick Sawyer. Wikipedia, The Free Encyclopedia. October 21, 2022, 14:02 UTC. https://en.wikipedia.org/w/index.php?title=Patrick _Sawyer&oldid=1117395418

4. Wilson J. Ebola fears hit close to home. CNN. https://www.cnn.com/2014/07 /29/health/ebola-outbreak-american-dies. Published July 30, 2014.

5. Ross W. Ebola crisis: How Nigeria's Dr Adadevoh fought the virus. BBC News. https://www.bbc.com/news/world-africa-29696011. Published October 20, 2014.

6. Daly M. How bureaucrats let Ebola spread to Nigeria. The Daily Beast. www .thedailybeast.com. Published April 14, 2014.

7. Ogunlesi T. Dr. Stella Ameyo Adadevo: Ebola victim and everyday hero. *The Guardian*. https://www.theguardian.com/lifeandstyle/womens-blog/2014/oct/20/dr -stella-ameyo-adadevoh-ebola-doctor-nigeria-hero. Published October 20, 2014. Accessed September 18, 2015.

8. "Nigeria: Tributes to Dr. Stella Ameyo Adadevo." August 26, 2014. https:// allafrica.com/stories/201408250338.html

9. Szabo L. Avoid non-essential travel to Ebola nations. *USA Today*. https://www .usatoday.com/story/news/nation/2014/07/31/cdc-ebola-travel-advisory/13413437/. Published/updated July 31, 2014.

10. Babatunde S. Flashback: 'Crazy Man' Patrick Sawyer brought Ebola to Nigeria three years ago. International Centre for Investigative Reporting. https://www .icirnigeria.org/flashback-crazy-man-patrick-sawyer-brought-ebola-to-nigeria-three -years-ago. Published July 25, 2017.

11. Porzuki N. Decontee Sawyer remembers the life of her husband—the First American victim of Ebola's latest outbreak. PRI's The World. https://theworld.org /stories/2014-08-01/decontee-sawyer-remembers-life-her-husband-first-american -victim-ebolas-latest. Published August 1, 2014.

12. Flashback: How Sawyer passed Ebola on to Dr. Ada Igonoh and how she survived. The Cable. https://www.thecable.ng/how-i-survived-ebola-2. Published July 20, 2015.

13. A report: Lessons learned from managing and coordinating the Ebola response in Liberia, Presidential Advisory Council on Ebola and the UN Resident Coordinator System in Liberia

14. Two Americans stricken with deadly Ebola virus in Liberia. NBC News. http://www.nbcnews.com/storyline/ebola-virus-outbreak/two-americans-stricken-deadly-ebola-virus-liberia-n166281. Published July 28, 2014.

15. Doucleff M. 2 Americans catch Ebola in Liberia. NPR. https://www.npr.org/sections/goatsandsoda/2014/07/28/336043452/2-americans-catch-ebola-in-liberia-as-nigeria-reports-first-case. Published July 28, 2014.

16. Botelho G, Brumfield B, Carter CJ. Two Americans infected with Ebola in Liberia coming to Atlanta hospital. CNN. https://www.cnn.com/2014/08/01/health/ebola-outbreak. Published August 2, 2014.

17. Two Americans who had been infected with Ebola leave Atlanta hospital. The Telegraph. https://www.telegraph.co.uk/news/worldnews/ebola/11049109/Two-Americans-who-had-been-infected-with-Ebola-leave-Atlanta-hospital.html. Published August 21, 2014.

18. Blinder A, Grady D. American doctor with Ebola arrives in US. *New York Times*. https://www.nytimes.com/2014/08/03/us/kent-brantley-nancy-writebol-ebola-treatment-atlanta.html. Published August 3, 2014.

19. Kassam A. Ebola: Spanish missionary infected with virus in Liberia flown to Spain. The Guardian. https://www.theguardian.com/world/2014/aug/07/ebola-spanish-missionary-miguel-pajares-virus-liberia-flown-spain. Published August 7, 2014.

20. Nyenswah TG, Kateh F, Bawo L, et al. Ebola and its control in Liberia, 2014–2015. *Emerg Infect Dis*. 2016;22(2):169–177. https://doi.org/10.3201/eid2202.151456

21. Liberian Institute of Statistics and Geo-Information Services, The World Bank Group. The Socio-Economic Impacts of Ebola in Liberia. April 15, 2015. https://www.worldbank.org/en/topic/poverty/publication/socio-economic-impacts-ebola-liberia

22. WHO, Ebola Situation Report April 8, 2015. http://apps.who.int/gho/data/view.ebola-sitrep.ebola-summary-latest?lang=eng

23. Investment plan for building a resilient health system 2015 to 2021. Ministry of Health, Government of Liberia. https://au.int/web/sites/default/files/newsevents/workingdocuments/27027-wd-liberia-_investment_plan_for_building_a_resilient_health_system.pdf

24. Liberia president declares Ebola curfew. Fox News. https://www.foxnews.com/health/liberia-president-declares-ebola-curfew. Published October 27, 2015.

25. Statement on the 9th meeting of the IHR Emergency Committee regarding the Ebola outbreak in West Africa. World Health Organization. https://www.who.int/news-room/detail/29-03-2016-statement-on-the-9th-meeting-of-the-ihr-emergency-committee-regarding-the-ebola-outbreak-in-west-africa. Published March 29, 2016.

26. Durrheim DN, Gostin LO, Moodley K. When does a major outbreak become a public health emergency of international Concern? *Lancet*. https://doi.org/10.1016/S1473-3099(20)30401-1

27. 2014–2016 Ebola outbreak in West Africa. CDC. https://www.cdc.gov/vhf/ebola/history/2014-2016-outbreak/index.html

28. UN Declares Ebola outbreak global 'international public health emergency.' UN News. Available at: https://news.un.org/en/story/2014/08/474732. Published August 8, 2014.

29. Epidemiological update: Outbreak of Ebola virus disease in West Africa, 21 August 2014. European Centre for Disease Prevention and Control. https://www.ecdc .europa.eu/en/news-events/epidemiological-update-outbreak-ebola-virus-disease -west-africa-21-august-2014

30. Botelho G, Wilson J. Thomas Eric Duncan: First Ebola death in U.S. CNN. https://www.cnn.com/2014/10/08/health/thomas-eric-duncan-ebola/index.html. Published October 8, 2014.

31. Fernandez M, Onishi N. U.S. patient aided Ebola victim in Liberia. *New York Times*. https://www.nytimes.com/2014/10/02/us/after-ebola-case-in-dallas-health -officials-seek-those-who-had-contact-with-patient.html. Published October 1, 2014.

32. Lupkin S. Ebola in America: Timeline of the deadly virus. How the Ebola virus came to the United States and spread. ABC News. https://abcnews.go.com/Health /ebola-america-timeline/story?id=26159719. Published November 17, 2014.

CHAPTER 4: A Refugee in Côte d'Ivoire

1. CDC director on Ebola: 'We are definitely not at the peak.' NPR: All Things Considered. https://www.npr.org/sections/goatsandsoda/2014/08/26/343436300 /cdc-director-on-ebola-we-are-definitely-not-at-the-peak. Published August 26, 2014.

2. Grady D. Ebola cases could reach 1.4 million within four months, CDC estimates. *New York Times*. https://www.nytimes.com/2014/09/24/health/ebola-cases-could -reach-14-million-in-4-months-cdc-estimates.html. Published September 23, 2014.

3. Lupkin S. Ebola could infect 1.4 million people by end of January, CDC projects. ABC News. https://abcnews.go.com/Health/ebola-infect-14-million-people -end-january-cdc/story?id=25698878. Published September 23, 2014.

4. Liberian human rights violator removed from US. US Immigration and Customs Enforcement. https://www.ice.gov/news/releases/liberian-human-rights -violator-removed-us. Published March 29, 2012.

CHAPTER 5: Total Collapse of Public Health Care Services

1. Republic of Liberia Investment Plan for Building a Resilient Health System in Liberia 2015 to 2021. https://au.int/web/sites/default/files/newsevents /workingdocuments/27027-wd-liberia-_investment_plan_for_building_a_resilient _health_system.pdf. Updated April 15, 2015.

2. Public Health Emergency, Emergency Management and Incident Command Systems. https://www.phe.gov/Preparedness/planning/mscc/handbook/aspx#1.3.2. Retrieved November 7, 2021.

3. Hessou C. Pregnant in the shadow of Ebola: Deteriorating health systems endanger women. United National Population Fund (UNFPA). https://www.unfpa .org/news/pregnant-shadow-ebola-deteriorating-health-systems-endanger-women. Published October 20, 2014.

4. Collins-Andrews B, McQuilkin P, Udhayashankar K, Adu E, Moormann A. Presentation and treatment outcomes of Liberian children age 5 years and under diagnosed with severe malaria. *Glob Pediatr Health*. 2019;6. https://doi.org/10.1177 /2333794X19884818

5. The President's Malaria Initiative. The White House. https://georgewbush-whitehouse.archives.gov/infocus/malaria/.

6. United Nations. Universal Declaration of Human Rights. Published 1948. https://www.un.org/en/about-us/universal-declaration-of-human-rights. Accessed November 7, 2021.

CHAPTER 6: Security Challenge

1. World Food Programme. WFP News Video Ebola: WFP delivering food in quarantine areas in Liberia. Location: Dolo's Town, Margibi County, Liberia. Filmed September 5, 2014. https://www.wfp.org/videos/ebola-wfp-delivering-food-quarantine-areas-liberia-media

2. Republic of Liberia Ministry of Health and Social Welfare. *National Health and Social Welfare Policy and Plan 2011–2021*, p. 18. https://moh.gov.lr/wp-content/uploads/National-Health-Policy-Plan-MOH-2011-2021.pdf

3. Associated Press. Liberia president declares Ebola curfew. Fox News. August 19, 2014. https://www.foxnews.com/health/liberia-president-declares-ebola-curfew

4. Federal Emergency Management Agency (FEMA). *National Incident Management System*, 3rd ed., p. 3. October 2017. Available at https://www.fema.gov/sites/default/files/2020-07/fema_nims_doctrine-2017.pdf

5. Special envoy on Ebola. Global Ebola Response. Retrieved November 7, 2021. https://ebolaresponse.un.org/special-envoy-ebola

6. Disease or condition of the week: Ebola—Key facts. US Centers for Disease Control and Prevention website. www.cdc.gov/dotw/ebola

7. Nyenswah TG, Kateh F, Bawo L, et. al. Ebola and its control in Liberia, 2014–2015. *Emerg Infect Dis.* 2016 Feb;22(2):169–77. https://www.ncbi.nlm.nih.gov/pmc/articles/PMC4734504/

8. Ebola virus disease—Democratic Republic of the Congo. World Health Organization website. https://www.who.int/emergencies/disease-outbreak-news/item/ebola-virus-disease-democratic-republic-of-the-congo_1. Published October 10, 2021.

9. Cameroonian doctor killed by rebels in DR Congo. *Journal du Cameroun.* https://www.journalducameroun.com/en/cameroonian-doctor-killed-by-rebels-in-dr-congo/. Published April 22, 2019.

10. Kirsch TD, Moseson H, Massaquoi M, et al. Impact of interventions and the incidence of Ebola virus disease in Liberia—implications for future epidemics. *Health Policy Plan.* 2017; 32(2):206 and 209–210. https://www.ncbi.nlm.nih.gov/pmc/articles/PMC6279138/pdf/czw113.pdf. Accessed November 7, 2021.

CHAPTER 7: Interventions

1. 2014 Ebola outbreak response—Ebola report: tracing contacts. US Centers for Disease Control and Prevention (CDC) website. https://www.cdc.gov/about/ebola/tracing-contacts.html. Accessed November 8, 2021.

2. Contact tracing in the context of COVID-19. Interim guidance, 10 May 2020. World Health Organization. https://www.who.int/csr/resources/publications/ebola/contact-tracing-during-outbreak-of-ebola.pdf

3. The Ebola outbreak in Liberia is over. WHO Africa Region. https://www.afro.who.int/news/ebola-outbreak-liberia-over. Published May 9, 2015.

4. MOHSW Situation Report, January 2015. Unpublished IMS presentation.

5. Fallah M, Dahn B, Nyenswah T, et al. Interrupting Ebola transmission in Liberia through community-based initiatives. *Ann Intern Med.* 2016;164:367–369. https://doi.org/10.7326/M15-1464

6. Peremans M, and Stockholm Evaluation Unit. OCB Ebola review—Part 4: Advocacy & communications. https://evaluation.msf.org/sites/default/files/attachments/ocb_evaluation_ebola_advocacy_final_0.pdf. Published February 2016.

7. MOHSW. *Situation Report, Mid-August 2014.* Unpublished IMS presentation.

8. MOHSW. *National Ebola Strategic Plan.* Unpublished government document.

9. US Public Health Service Commission Corps. Monrovia Medical Unit (Ebola Treatment Unit). https://pahx.org/wp-content/uploads/2016/11/Corps-MMU-ETU_Overview-Nov-7_2014_Final.pdf

10. Kateh F, Nagbe T, Kieta A, et al. Rapid response to Ebola outbreaks in remote areas—Liberia, July–November 2014. *Morbidity and Mortality Weekly Report.* 2015;64(7):188–192. https://www.cdc.gov/mmwr/preview/mmwrhtml/mm6407a7.htm?s_cid=mm6407a7_w

11. Liberia Institute of Statistics and Geo-Information Services (LISGIS), Ministry of Health [Liberia], and ICF. *Liberia: Demographic and Health Survey 2019–20.* Liberia Institute of Statistics and Geo-Information Services (LISGIS), Ministry of Health, and ICF; 2021. https://dhsprogram.com/pubs/pdf/FR362/FR362.pdf

12. Community mobilization: Essential for stopping the spread of Ebola. Mercy Corps. Version 1.0, May 29, 2019. https://www.mercycorps.org/sites/default/files/2020-01/CommunityMobilizationEbola-May29-FINAL.pdf

13. Schreiber L. "Everybody's business": Mobilizing citizens during Liberia's Ebola outbreak, 2014–2015. Innovations for Successful Societies, Princeton University; 2017.

14. Republic of Liberia, Incident Management System. *Guide for Religious Leaders Prevention & Control Ebola Virus Disease.* September 2015. Unpublished government document.

15. Lev. 13:1. https://kingjames.bible/Leviticus-13#1

16. Lev. 13:2. https://kingjames.bible/Leviticus-13#2

17. IREX: A global development & education organization. https://www.irex.org/

18. Broadhurst MJ, Brooks TJG, Pollock NR. Diagnosis of Ebola virus disease: Past, present, and future. *Clin Microbiol Rev.* 2016;29(4):773–793. https://doi.org/10.1128/CMR.00003-16

19. Office of the UN Secretary-General's Special Envoy on Ebola and Multi-Partner Trust Fund Office, UNDP. *Interim Report for the period October 2014 to January 2015* [pre-publication version]. https://ebolaresponse.un.org/sites/default/files/mptf_report20022015final_0.pdf

20. Nyenswah T. Ebola outbreak response Liberia, December 19, 2014, page 18. Unpublished presentation.

21. Empowering communities to conduct safe burial practices. WHO Africa. https://www.afro.who.int/news/empowering-communities-conduct-safe-burial -practices. Published March 20, 2015.

22. Jallah JD. Unpublished presentation to APORA Conference, Farmington Hotel, Margibi County, November 13, 2018.

23. Ministry of Health, Miatta Z. Gbanya, deputy incident manager. Ebola Response / MOH on behalf of the Human Resource Team (MOH/PFMU/MoFDP), an unpublished presentation on Hazard Pay, April 14, 2015.

24. GoL payroll status, NGO employment, Hazard pay. PACE decision briefing on Health Worker Compensation. October 24, 2014. Unpublished presentation.

25. Ebola: World Bank Group approves US$105 million grant for faster epidemic containment in Guinea, Liberia, and Sierra Leone. World Bank website. https://www .worldbank.org/en/news/press-release/2014/09/16/ebola-world-bank-group -approves-grant-faster-epidemic-containment-guinea-liberia-sierra-leone. Published September 16, 2014.

26. Liberia's 168th independence anniversary kicks off with investiture ceremony; 42 honored, eight, deceased healthcare workers posthumously. https://www.emansion .gov.lr/2press.php?news_id=3355&related=7&pg=sp. Published July 17, 2015.

CHAPTER 8: The International Response

1. Biosecurity. Department of Agriculture, Environment and Rural Affairs (DAERA). https://www.daera-ni.gov.uk/articles/biosecurity. Published March 4, 2022.

2. Strengthening health security across the globe: Progress and impact of U.S. government investments in the Global Health Security Agenda. Global Healthy Security Agenda 2020 annual report. https://www.whitehouse.gov/wp-content /uploads/2021/10/Global-Health-Security-Agenda-Annual-Report.pdf

3. Katz R, Sorrell EM, Kornblet SA, et al. Global health security agenda and the international health regulations: Moving forward. *Biosecur Bioterror*. 2014;12(5): 231–238.

4. World Health Organization (WHO). Implementation of the international health regulations (2005) 2016; A69/21.

5. Advancing the global health security agenda: Progress and early impact from U.S. investment. Global Health Security Agenda 2016 annual report 2016. https:// www.state.gov/wp-content/uploads/2019/02/1-ghsa-annual-report-2016.pdf

6. Ebola virus disease: Overview. World Health Organization website. https:// www.who.int/health-topics/ebola#tab=tab_1

7. 2014 Ebola virus outbreak: Facts, symptoms, and how to help. World Vision website. https://www.worldvision.org/health-news-stories/2014-ebola-virus -outbreak-facts

8. Liberia's Ellen Johnson Sirleaf urges world help on Ebola. BBC News. https:// www.bbc.com/news/world-africa-29680934. Published October 19, 2014.

9. Ebola: Liberia's president pens heartfelt letter to the world. Opinion Nigeria website. https://www.opinionnigeria.com/ebola-liberias-president-pens-heartfelt -letter-to-the-world/. Published October 19, 2014.

10. Ebola outbreak: WHO warns that virus could infect 20,000. BBC News. https://www.bbc.com/news/world-africa-28971710. Published August 28, 2014.

11. Ebola virus disease, 2014–2016 Ebola outbreak in West Africa. Centers for Disease Control and Prevention website. https://www.cdc.gov/vhf/ebola/history /2014-2016-outbreak/index.html

12. The African Union response to EVD outbreak in West Africa; AU deployment diagram. https://www.un.org/en/ecosoc/ebola1/pdf/au_ebola_timeline.pdf

13. This Congolese doctor discovered Ebola but never got credit for it—until now (NPR). University of Washington Department of Global Health. https://globalhealth .washington.edu/news/2019/11/07/congolese-doctor-discovered-ebola-never-got -credit-it-until-now-npr-includes-peter. Published November 7, 2019.

14. The Congolese doctor who discovered Ebola. National Public Radio. https:// www.npr.org/2020/07/08/889008647/the-congolese-doctor-who-discovered-ebola. Broadcast July 9, 2020.

15. Democratic Republic of Congo profile—Timeline. May 4, 2011. A chronology of key events: Rule of the Kabilas. https://www.bbc.com/news/world-africa-13286306

16. West Africa Ebola Outbreak—Fact Sheet #1 August 14, 2014. USAID. https://www.usaid.gov/fact-sheet/west-africa-ebola-outbreak-fact-sheet-1

17. Mason JL. Operation United Assistance during the Ebola outbreak in West Africa in 2014–2015. https://history.army.mil/covid19/History-Op-UNITED-ASSISTANCE.pdf

18. Operation United Assistance: The DOD response to Ebola in West Africa. Joint and Coalition Operational Analysis. https://www.jcs.mil/Portals/36 /Documents/Doctrine/ebola/OUA_report_jan2016.pdf. Published January 6, 2016.

19. West Africa—Ebola outbreak. Fact Sheet #9, fiscal year 2016. USAID. https://www.usaid.gov/sites/default/files/documents/1866/west_africa_ebola_fs09 _03-24-2016.pdf. Published March 24, 2016.

20. Mobula LM, Nakao JH, Walia S, et al. A humanitarian response to the West Africa Ebola virus disease outbreak. *J Int. Humanit. Action.* 2018;3(10). https://doi .org/10.1186/s41018-018-0039-2

21. PHEP operational readiness review. CDC website. https://www.cdc.gov/cpr /readiness/mcm-readiness.html#. Last reviewed May 13, 2022.

22. National Institute of Health and Government of Liberia. *Partnership for Research on Ebola Virus in Liberia (PREVAIL), Strategic Plan 2016–2021.* Unpublished.

23. Ebola virus disease. World Health Organization website. http://who.int /mediacentre/factsheets/fs103/en/. Published February 23, 2021.

24. Kennedy SB, Bolay F, Kieh, M, et al. Phase 2 placebo-controlled trial of two vaccines to prevent Ebola in Liberia. *N Engl J Med* 2017; 377:1438–1447. https://doi .org/10.1056/NEJMoa1614067. Published October 12, 2017.

25. Ebola outbreak in DRC: Second-largest outbreak in history rages in Congo. Concern Worldwide US. https://www.concernusa.org/story/ebola-outbreak-in-drc/. Published January 11, 2020.

26. WHO declares an end to second Ebola outbreak in Guinea. Agence France-Press. https://www.voanews.com/a/africa_who-declares-end-second-ebola-outbreak -guinea/6207223.html. Published June 19, 2021.

27. Marston BJ, Dokubo E, van Steelandt A, et al. Ebola response impact on public health programs, West Africa, 2014–2017. *Emerg Infect Dis*. 2017;23(13). https://doi.org/10.3201/eid2313.170727

28. Peremans M, and Stockholm Evaluation Unit. OCB Ebola review—Part 4: Advocacy & communications. https://evaluation.msf.org/sites/default/files /attachments/ocb_evaluation_ebola_advocacy_final_0.pdf. Published February 2016.

29. Update: Ebola virus disease outbreak—West Africa, October 2014. *Morbidity and Mortality Weekly Report*. 2014. 63(43);978–981. https://www.cdc.gov/mmwr /preview/mmwrhtml/mm6343a3.htm#:~:text=According%20to%20the%20latest%20 World%20Health%20Organization%20update,West%20African%20countries%20 %28Guinea%2C%20Liberia%2C%20and%20Sierra%20Leone%29

30. MOH Sitrep #156. Unpublished report from EPI Bulletin.

31. MSF France Inpatient Facility Proposal. Monrovia, Liberia; October 2014. Ministry of Health archives.

32. National Incident Management Team meeting minutes, 8/28/2014.

33. The role of WHO within the United Nations Mission for Ebola Emergency Response. World Health Organization website. https://www.who.int/publications/m /item/the-role-of-who-within-the-united-nations-mission-for-ebola-emergency -response. Published April 1, 2015.

34. Resolution 69/1: Measures to contain and combat the recent Ebola outbreak in West Africa. United Nations General Assembly. https://www.un.org/en/ga/view _doc.asp?symbol=A/RES/69/1. Published September 23, 2014.

35. Resolution 2177: Peace and Security in Africa. United Nations Security Council. Published September 18, 2014.

36. United Nations Mission for Ebola Emergency Response. World Health Organization website. https://www.who.int/csr/resources/publications/ebola/who-unmeer/en/

37. Unicef-Liberia, Ebola Virus Disease: SitRep #48, 22 August 2014. https:// reliefweb.int/sites/reliefweb.int/files/resources/pdf

38. EU response to Ebola: Factsheet. European Commission website. opa.eu https://civil-protection-humanitarian-aid.ec.europa.eu/where/africa/eu-response -ebola_en

39. Sendolo J. Liberia: "We are here to build and maintain treatment/training centers"—Chinese ambassador declares as China invests U.S.$82 million in Ebola fight. Embassy of the People's Republic of Chine in the Republic of South Africa website. http://za.china-embassy.gov.cn/eng/zt/20141006b/201410/t20141028 _7635480.htm. Published October 28, 2014.

40. Tan Y, Wang X. China army medics join Ebola battle. *China Daily*. https://www .chinadaily.com.cn/china/2014-11/15/content_18918365.htm. Published November 15, 2014.

41. Huang Y. China's response to the 2014 Ebola outbreak in West Africa. *Glob Chall*. 2017;1(2):160001. https://doi.org/10.1002/gch2.201600001

42. Giahyue JH. Cuban doctors, nurses land in Liberia to fight Ebola alongside U.S. Reuters. https://www.reuters.com/article/us-heath-ebola-liberia -idUSKCN0IB1A520141022. Published October 22, 2014.

43. Chaple EB, Mercer MA. The Cuban response to the Ebola epidemic in West Africa: Lessons in Solidarity. *Int J Health Serv*. 2017, December;47(1):134–149. https://doi.org/10.1177/0020731416681892

44. Neal A. CNN documentary *Unseen Enemy* is terrifying look at human vulnerability in face of pandemics. Monsters & Critics website. https://www.monstersandcritics.com/tv/cnn-documentary-unseen-enemy-is-terrifying-look-at-human-vulnerability-in-face-of-pandemics/. Published April 7, 2017.

45. Liberia: Germany to provide logistical help to Ebola-hit Liberia. All Africa. https://allafrica.com/stories/201409180250.html. Published September 17, 2014.

46. Chancellor Merkel says Germany will provide logistical help to tackle Ebola crisis in Liberia. Associated Press/New Europe. https://www.neweurope.eu/article/chancellor-merkel-says-germany-will-provide-logistical-help-tackle-ebola-crisis-liberia/. Published September 17, 2014.

47. Janke C, Heim KM, Steiner F, et al. Beyond Ebola treatment units: Severe infection temporary treatment units as an essential element of Ebola case management during an outbreak. *BMC Infect Dis*. 2017;17(1):124. https://www.ncbi.nlm.nih.gov/pmc/articles/PMC5295220/pdf/12879_2017_Article_2235.pdf

48. Nyenswah T, Engineer CY, Peters DH. Leadership in times of crisis: The example of Ebola virus disease in Liberia. *Health Syst Reform*. 2016, July 2;2(3):194–207. https://doi.org/10.1080/23288604.2016.1222793

49. World Bank Group approves US$285 million grant for ongoing Ebola crisis response. World Bank website. https://www.worldbank.org/en/news/press-release/2014/11/18/world-bank-group-grant-ongoing-ebola-crisis-response. Published November 18, 2014.

50. Restructuring paper on a proposed project restructuring of Ebola Emergency Response Project approved on September 16, 2014, to Republic of Liberia, Republic of Sierra Leone, Republic of Guinea. The World Bank. Ebola Emergency Response Project (P152359). https://documents1.worldbank.org/curated/en/494061576852002648/pdf/Disclosable-Restructuring-Paper-Ebola-Emergency-Response-Project-P152359.pdf

51. Croft A. Ebola-hit countries seek help to repair their economies. Reuters. https://www.reuters.com/article/us-health-ebola-conference/ebola-hit-countries-seek-help-to-repair-their-economies-idINKBN0LZ1VS20150304. Published March 4, 2015.

52. Logistics and capacity development support for the humanitarian Community's response to the Ebola virus disease outbreak in Libera (Operation ID: 200926). World Food Programme. https://www.wfp.org/operations/200926-logistics-and-capacity-development-support-humanitarian-communitys-response-ebola

CHAPTER 9: Recovery, Rebuilding, and Resiliency

1. 2014–2016 Ebola outbreak in West Africa. Centers for Disease Control and Prevention website. https://www.cdc.gov/vhf/ebola/history/2014-2016-outbreak/index.html. Published March 8, 2019.

2. Latest Ebola outbreak over in Liberia; West Africa is at zero, but flare-ups are likely to occur. World Health Organization website. https://www.who.int/news/item

/14-01-2016-latest-ebola-outbreak-over-in-liberia-west-africa-is-at-zero-but-new -flare-ups-are-likely-to-occur. Published January 14, 2016.

3. Investment Plan for Building a Resilient Health System 2015 to 2021. Ministry of Health, Government of Liberia. https://moh.gov.lr/documents/policy/2020 /investment-plan-for-building-a-resilient-health-system/. Published May 12, 2015.

4. Agenda for transformation: Steps towards Liberia RISING 2030. https:// allafrica.com/download/resource/main/main/idatcs/00080846:1b0f1d46c3e2c30c516 58f7f64dcb7b9.pdf

5. Manyazewal T. Using the World Health Organization health system building blocks through survey of healthcare professionals to determine the performance of public healthcare facilities. *Arch Public Health*. 2017;75:50. https://doi.org/10.1186 /s13690-017-0221-9

6. Monitoring the building blocks of health systems: A handbook of indicators and their measurement strategies. World Health Organization; 2010:8–10. https:// apps.who.int/iris/bitstream/handle/10665/258734/9789241564052-eng.pdf

7. Kluge H, Martín-Moreno JM, Emiroglu N, et al. Strengthening global health security by embedding the International Health Regulations requirements into national health systems. *BMJ Glob Health* 2018;3:e000656. https://doi.org/10.1136 /bmjgh-2017-000656

8. Ebola transmission in Liberia over. Nation enters 90-day intensive surveillance period. World Health Organization website. https://www.who.int/news/item /03-09-2015-ebola-transmission-in-liberia-over-nation-enters-90-day-intensive -surveillance-period. Published September 3, 2015.

9. WHO declares the end of the most recent Ebola virus disease outbreak in Liberia. https://www.afro.who.int/news/who-declares-end-most-recent-ebola-virus -disease-outbreak-liberia-0. Published June 9, 2016.

10. Health Communication Capacity Collaborative. *Social mobilization lessons learned: The Ebola response in Liberia*. Johns Hopkins Center for Communication Programs; February 2017. https://healthcommcapacity.org/wp-content/uploads/2017 /02/Ebola-Lessons-Learned-ksm.pdf

11. Ministry of Health National Public Health Institute of Liberia, World Health Organization, and US Centers for Disease Control and Prevention. National Technical Guidelines for Integrated Disease Surveillance & Response. https:// reliefweb.int/report/liberia/ministry-health-and-national-public-health-institute -liberia-national-technical. Published September 13, 2021.

12. Public Health Agency Canada. A report of the National Advisory Committee on SARS and Public Health October 2003, Learning from SARS, Renewal of Public Health Canada. https://www.canada.ca/content/dam/phac-aspc/migration/phac -aspc/publicat/sars-sras/pdf/sars-e.pdf

13. CDC. The U.S. Public Health Service and Malaria 1914–1942. https://www.cdc .gov/malaria/about/history/index.html

14. Twelfth Report: Public Health. House of Commons. Health Committee. October 19, 2011. https://en.wikipedia.org/wiki/Public_Health_England#cite_note -:1-1. Retrieved November 8, 2021.

15. African Union. Africa CDC. About us. https://africacdc.org/about-us/our-history/

16. Kennedy SB, Bolay F, Kieh M, et al. Phase 2 placebo-controlled trial of two vaccines to prevent Ebola in Liberia. *N Engl J Med.* 2017;377(15):1438–1447. https://doi.org/10.1056/NEJMoa1614067

17. Intergovernmental Personnel Act (IPA) mobility program. National Institute of Health, Office of Human Resources. https://hr.nih.gov/workforce/ipa

18. Peters DH, Hanssen O, Gutierrez J, Abrahams J, Nyenswah T. Financing common goods for health: Core government functions in health emergency and disaster risk management. *Health Syst Reform.* 2019;5(4):307–321. https://doi.org/10.1080/23288604.2019

19. Nyenswah T, Engineer CY, Peters DH. Leadership in times of crisis: The example of Ebola virus disease in Liberia. *Health Syst Reform.* 2016;2(3):194–207. https://doi.org/10.1080/23288604.2016.1222793

20. Global Health Security Index. https://www.ghsindex.org/

21. Shamasunder S, Holmes SM. COVID-19 reveals weak health systems by design: Why we must re-make global health in this historic moment. *Glob Public Health.* 2020;15(7):1083–1089. https://doi.org/10.1080/17441692.2020.1760915

22. Quick JD, Fryer B. *The End of Epidemics: The Looming Threat to Humanity and How to Stop It.* St. Martin's Press; 2018:108–109.

23. Pearce K. Johns Hopkins launches online course to train army of contact tracers to slow spread of COVID-19. Johns Hopkins University. https://hub.jhu.edu/2020/05/11/free-contact-tracing-course-johns-hopkins/. Published May 11, 2020.

24. Gurley E. COVID-19 contract tracing. Coursera online course. https://www.coursera.org/learn/covid-19-contact-tracing?edocomorp=covid-19-contact-tracing

25. Kruk M, Myers M, Varpilah T, et al. What is a resilient health system? Lessons from Ebola. *Lancet.* 2015;385(9980):1910–1912. https://doi.org/10.1016/s0140-6736(15)60755-3

26. Nyenswah T. Leadership in times of crisis: A personal reflection from the center of the Ebola epidemic response in Liberia. *Health Syst Reform.* 2016;2(3):208–212. https://doi.org/10.1080/23288604.2016.1216253

CHAPTER 10: Reflections

1. Sirleaf EJ. Text of Ellen Johnson Sirleaf's speech. *Harvard Gazette.* https://news.harvard.edu/gazette/story/2011/05/text-of-ellen-johnson-sirleafs-speech/. Published May 26, 2011.

2. Zagursky R. Do owners/CEOs only hear what they want to hear or listen to what they need to hear? Assured Strategy. https://www.assuredstrategy.com/do-ownersceos-only-hear-what-they-want-to-hear-or-listen-to-what-they-need-to-hear-by-rony-zagursky/. Published July 20, 2015.

3. Fubini D. *Hidden Truths: What Leaders Need to Hear But Are Rarely Told.* John Wiley & Sons; 2021:166.

4. Nyenswah T. Leadership in times of crisis: A personal reflection from the center of the Ebola epidemic response in Liberia. *Health Syst Reform.* 2016;2(3):208–212. https://doi.org/10.1080/23288604.2016.1216253

5. The United Nations Human Settlements Programme (UN-Habitat). Social Mobilization https://www.fukuoka.unhabitat.org/docs/publications/pdf/peoples _process/ChapterII-Social_Mobilization.pdf

6. National Public Health Institute of Liberia. Situation Report: Confirmed COVID-19. https://www.nphil.gov.lr/wp-content/uploads/2020/10/LR-COVID-19 -Situation-Report-01-March-16-2020.pdf. Published March 16, 2020.

7. Nyenswah TG, Kateh F, Bawo L, et. al. Ebola and its control in Liberia, 2014– 2015. *Emerg Infect Dis*. 2016;22(2):169–177. https://doi.org/10.3201/eid2202.151456

8. This Congolese doctor discovered Ebola but never got the credit—until now (NPR). University of Washington Department of Global Health. https://globalhealth .washington.edu/news/2019/11/07/congolese-doctor-discovered-ebola-never-got -credit-it-until-now-npr-includes-peter. Published November 7, 2019.

9. The discovery of and research on the Ebola virus. Institute of Tropical Medicine, Antwerp. https://www.itg.be/E/the-discovery-of-and-research-on-the -ebola-virus. Published November 1, 2022.

10. Paoli J. Viruses 101: What's multiplying in you? Scitable by Nature Education. https://www.nature.com/scitable/blog/viruses101/the_scientist_who_discovered _ebola/. Published November 5, 2014.

11. Clark L. A new beginning—Liberia Marathon 2015. Medium.com. https:// medium.com/@larissaclark/a-new-beginning-is-the-theme-of-the-2015-liberia -marathon-which-will-take-place-on-sunday-34ebe3a2f0a8. Published July 16, 2015.

12. Liberia Marathon Facebook page. November 8, 2015. https://www.facebook .com/LiberiaMarathon/posts/935152206559026

13. Liberia National Anthem lyrics. Lyrics on Demand website. https://www .lyricsondemand.com/miscellaneouslyrics/nationalanthemslyrics/liberianational anthemlyrics.html

achekeh, 67
Action Aid, 176
active case finding: as basic to control, 108; challenges in, 113; and early responses, 93, 95; and IMS, 108, 111–15, 121. *See also* contact tracing
Adadevoh, Ameyo Stella, 42
Adventist Development and Relief Agency (ADRA), 56, 62, 63
Africa Centres for Disease Control and Prevention (ACDC), 144, 145–47, 185
African Field Epidemiology Training Network, 186
African scientists: recognition of, xvi–xvii, 145, 204–8; and research paper credit, 196–97
African Union (AU), xiv, 24, 104, 144–47, 161, 165
African Union Support to Ebola in West Africa (ASEOWA), xiv, 144–45, 161
Africare, 174
Agenda for Transformation (AFT), 181
Aggor, Divine, 34
aid. *See* funding and aid
AIDS/HIV, 87, 90, 129
airlines and air transport: and COVID-19, 202; Ebola screenings, 138, 203; stoppages, 3, 43, 138
Americo-Liberians, 31, 32
Angie Brooks Randell, 174
animation cells, 130
Annan, Kofi, 86
antibodies, 9
ASEOWA (African Union Support to Ebola in West Africa), xiv, 144–45, 161
Aylward, Bruce, 107, 142, 158

Baawo, Saye, 80
Banbury, Anthony, 107
Bartee, Nathaniel, 84
Bawo, Luke, 119–22
Bayiah, Alex, 59
Beard-Beard, 57–59
Bennett, Sara, 187
Berg Report, 24
Bill & Melinda Gates Foundation, 160
Bin, Li, 163
biobank, 183
bleeding, as symptom, 8, 9, 10
Bloomberg Philanthropies, 190
Boakai, Joseph, 177
Bolay, Fatoma, 152
Boley, George, 51–52
borders: closing of, 6, 15, 47, 131; cross-border agreement, 44; screenings at, 138, 173, 174; and transmission, 9–10, 15
Brantley, Kent, x–xi, 44–45
brincidofovir, 48
Brisbane, Samuel, 44
Broh, Mary, 171, 193
Brown, Jerry, 12
Brown, Lewis, 171–72
Brussels Airlines, 138
Bryant, Charles Gyude, 84
building blocks framework, 181–82
Bundibugyo ebolavirus, 8
Burwell, Sylvia, 152
Bush, George W., 87

cAd3-EBOZ vaccine, 153, 186
Callaghan, Tim, 160
CARE International, 174
Carter Center, 174

case management: data challenges, 13; and
IMS, xiii, 103, 106, 108, 112, 115–19, 125;
international support for, 142, 151, 173,
174; and psychosocial support, 132
cemeteries, 39–40, 132, 133, 134
Center for Public Health Law Program,
184
Centers for Disease Control and Prevention (CDC): and COVID-19, 190, 202–3;
experience with Ebola, 139; and IMS,
75–77, 91, 101, 102, 104, 109; initial
response, 15; and malaria, 87, 185; and
National Public Health Institute of
Liberia, 184, 186; projections by, 4,
49–50; public health surveillance course,
88; and recovery efforts, 178; support
overview, xv, 147, 148, 150, 151, 159; and
testing, 131; travel warnings by, 3, 43;
visits by, 15, 43, 49, 147, 148; and Western
evacuees, 44
Chan, Margaret, 43–44, 47, 158, 163
China: and Tolbert Nyenswah, 24; support
from, xiv–xv, 161–63
CIA (Central Intelligence Agency), 25
civil society: and building resilience, 181;
criticism of response, 153; support from,
104, 174, 176
civil unrest: at government response, 14,
189; Rice Riots, 22–23, 25; and West
Point quarantine, xi–xii, 94–99
civil wars, 10–11, 35, 49, 50–58, 60, 83–84.
See also Nyenswah, Tolbert Geewleh, as
refugee
Clement, Peter, 144
Clinton, Bill, 174
Clinton Health Access Initiative (CHAI),
174
communication and messaging: and
community-based initiative, 114–15; on
funeral and burial practices, x, 37–38,
123, 155–56; and IMS, 106, 114–15, 123–
30; international support for, 128, 155,
159, 173–76; lack of community engagement in initial messaging, 14; and media, 125, 129–30, 172–73; technology, 104,
115, 121–22, 128; on touching, 18–19, 129
community-based initiative (CBI), 113–15
community care centers (CCCs), 118

community engagement: and ASEOWA,
145; and building resiliency, 182; challenges in, 125–26, 127; and contact
tracing, 113–15; and COVID-19, 201, 202,
203; importance of, 199–200, 203; and
IMS, xiv, 99, 103, 108, 113–15, 123–30;
lack of in initial response, xii, 14, 95–96,
114; and malaria, 87; and messaging,
124–27; need for, 98–99, 100; and NGOs,
173–76; and recovery, xv, 183; and vaccine trials, 153; and WHO, 144. *See also*
communication and messaging; social
mobilization
Community Health Assistance Program
(CHAP), 141
community health workers (CHWs), 18,
141, 159, 186
computer literacy, 82
Condé, Alpha, 147, 169
contact tracing: challenges in, 113; and
COVID-19, 188, 190–91, 201, 202, 203;
defined, 111; and IMS, xiii, 103, 105, 108,
111–15; and initial response, 3, 18, 95;
international support for, 144, 145, 169,
174, 175; in Nigeria, 42; and recovery, xv;
in West Point slum, 95
Cooper, Aloysius J., 38
Cooper, Nadu, 118–19
corpses: cremation of, x, 41–42, 133, 157;
dead body management and IMS, xiv,
103, 108, 109, 112, 116, 132–34; Dead
Body Management Team, x, 38–42; and
Red Cross, 15, 132–33; secret burials of,
x, 38, 42; in streets, x, 14, 38, 93, 96; and
transmission, x, 7, 11, 37–38, 132, 199–200.
See also funeral and burial practices
county health officers, 106
county health teams, 118
county operations and IMS, 103, 105–7, 118
coups: fear of, 148, 149; in 1980, 23
COVID-19 pandemic, 126, 186, 188–91, 198,
200–204
cremation, x, 41–42, 133, 157
Cuba, support from, xiv, 164–66
Cuevavirus, 8
Cull, Ellen, 184
curfews: national, xi, xii, 16, 47, 98; in West
Point, 95, 96

Dahn, Bernice: and Africa Centres for Disease Control and Prevention, 145, 147; and Ebola treatment units, 12; and IMS, 1, 76–77, 79–80, 103; and Médecins Sans Frontières, 15; and National Public Health Institute of Liberia, 183; and nomination of Tolbert Nyenswah as assistant minister, 90; and Presidential Task Force on Ebola, 16; and recovery, 179; and West Point quarantine, 95

data management: and building resiliency, 180, 181; challenges, 13; and community engagement, 125; and IMS, 105, 119–23, 125

Dead Body Management Team, x, 38–42

deaths: from civil unrest, xii, 98; from civil wars, 11, 49; from COVID-19, 201; from Ebola, ix, 5, 9, 141, 142, 155, 156, 194; and fatality rates, 8, 117, 120, 141; of health care workers, 13, 77, 164

De Cock, Kevin, 15, 75–76, 91, 102, 148

Democratic Republic of the Congo (DRC), outbreaks in, 13, 109–10, 154–55

Disaster Assistance Response Team (DART), 104, 147, 149–51, 160

disaster preparedness, 141, 171, 183

Disco Hill Cemetery, 133–34

Disease Prevention Division of MOHSW, 9, 17

distrust: and community engagement by IMS, 114, 123–24; and COVID-19 pandemic, 188; in government response, 14, 44, 123–24, 189; and hazard pay, 168; of health care system, x, 77, 178, 180; and PREVAIL, 153; and West Point security issues, 94, 95, 114

Doctors Without Borders. See Médecins Sans Frontières

Doe, Samuel Kanyon, 23, 25, 26, 50

Dolo's Town, 92, 95

Dukuly, Morris, 39

Duncan, Jesse, 90

Duncan, Thomas Eric, 48

Early Warning, Alert and Response Network (EWARN), 182, 183

Ebola Community Action Platform (ECAP), 127–29

Ebola fever. See Ebola virus disease

Ebola Fund, 194

Ebola Message Guide, 173

"Ebola Must Go, It's Everybody's Business" campaign, 125, 129

Ebola Survivor's Clinic, 165

Ebola treatment units (ETUs): admittance rates, 117, 119–20; challenges of, 115–16, 149–50, 167; and community engagement, 128–29; and dead body management, 40, 116; ELWA, 12, 15, 116, 156; fatality rates in, 117, 120; and feedback telephone system, 131–32; for health care workers, 117–18; IMS focus on, 108, 112–13, 115–19; international support for, xiv, 12, 15, 115–16, 148–50, 155–58, 162–63, 165–66, 169, 175; and Médecins Sans Frontières, xiv, 15, 115–16, 150, 155, 156–58; numbers of, 12, 96, 116–18; site selection for, 109, 150, 165; and SITTUs, 166–67

Ebolavirus, 8

Ebola virus disease (EVD): and antibodies, 9; discovery of, xvii, 8, 145, 204; fatality rates, 8, 117, 120, 141; incubation period, 8, 108, 111; lack of experience with, 10, 120, 139–40, 196; names for, 8; reporting obligations, 6–7; symptoms of, 8–9, 10; taxonomy of, 8; vaccines, 2, 7, 152–55, 186–87. See also medications; transmission; treatment

Ebola virus disease epidemic (2014–2016): case counts, ix, 45, 118, 119, 141, 156; deaths, ix, 5, 9, 141, 142, 155, 156, 194; end of declaration, xvii, 141, 177–78; fatality rates, 8, 117, 120, 141; first cases, 6–7, 9, 11; and later outbreaks, 178; lessons learned, xvi, 194–204; pause in, 37. See also communication and messaging; Ebola treatment units; funeral and burial practices; incident management system; international responses and support; isolation; social mobilization; transmission; treatment

Economic Community of West African States (ECOWAS), xiv, 143, 177

economics: and Berg Report, 24; costs of epidemic, 45, 170; effects on and fears

economics (*cont.*)
   for, 19, 45, 168, 169–70; GDP of Liberia,
   10; and Lagos Plan of Action, 24; and
   school closings, 170, 199
Economist Intelligence Unit, 188
Elder, Christian, 186
elections, 198
electricity, 78, 81
ELWA (Eternal Love Winning Africa), 12,
   15, 40, 116, 156
Emergency Ebola Response Project (EERP),
   136, 168–69
emergency preparedness, 3, 141, 171, 183
Emergency Preparedness and Response,
   171
Emergency Response Coordination Centre
   (European Union), 160
Emory University, 88
Epidemic Preparedness and Response plan,
   141, 182, 183, 201
Eternal Love Winning Africa (ELWA), 12,
   15, 40, 116, 156
ethnic conflict, 52
ETUs. *See* Ebola treatment units
European Centre for Disease Prevention
   and Control, 160
European Civil Protection and Humanitar-
   ian Aid Operations (ECHO), 161
European Union, support overview, xv,
   160–61
evacuations of Westerners, x–xi, 2, 42–43,
   44–45, 48, 116, 140, 175
Expanded Programme on Immunization
   (EPI), 90, 142

Fallah, Mosoka, 113
farming, 29–30, 51, 58–59
Fauci, Anthony, 184, 186
Fayiah, Comfort, 78
Fayiah, Victor, 78
feedback loop telephone system, 131–32
fever, 9, 10
field epidemiology program (FETP), 183
Filoviridae, 8
fishing, 54, 92
Flomo, Matthew T. K., 39
food: *achekeh*, 67; and nutritional support
   for Ebola, 103, 118–19; and quarantines,

95; and refugees, 54, 55, 56, 58, 61, 62, 70;
   and Rice Riots, 22–23, 25; and second
   civil war, 84; and UNICEF, 159; and
   World Bank, 169
Friday, Kiyee, 38
Frieden, Tom, 43, 49, 147
Fubini, David, 194
funding and aid: and building resiliency,
   182; and CBI volunteers, 114, 115–16;
   from China, 162, 163; estimates of, 195;
   from EU, 160–61; foreign aid as initially
   limited, 46, 116–17; of hazard pay, 136,
   168, 169; and National Public Health
   Institute of Liberia, 184, 185, 186; and
   Presidential Task Force on Ebola, 14, 16;
   and state-owned enterprises, 184; stolen
   and misused, 105; and surveillance
   challenges, 121; and UN, xv, 195; by US,
   151; for vaccine trials, 154; and WHO,
   143; and World Bank, xv, 136, 167–70
funeral and burial practices: community
   engagement on, 123, 125, 127, 129,
   199–200; and cremation, x, 41–42, 133,
   157; dead body management and IMS,
   xiv, 103, 108, 109, 112, 116, 132–34; Dead
   Body Management Team, x, 38–42;
   funeral of grandmother, 28–29; international support for, 169, 173, 175; and
   mass graves, 23; messaging on, x, 37–38,
   123, 155–56; and secret burials, x, 38, 42;
   and transmission, x, 7, 11, 37–38, 132,
   199–200; and West Point slum, 95

Gasasira, Alex, 46, 142, 158, 184
Gbanya, Miatta, 102–3, 135, 137
Gbowee, Leymah, 174
Gbowee Peace Foundation Africa (GPFA),
   174
gender: gender equity, 87; and literacy
   rates, 10, 124
General Services Agency (GSA), 171
German Red Cross, 167
Germany, support from, 166–67
Ghebreyesus, Tedros Adhanom, 110
Global Communities, 132–33
Global Fund, 86
Global Health Security Agenda (GHSA),
   140–41

Global Health Security Index (GHSI), 188
Gnassingbé, Faure, 177
gold, 51, 57, 59
Gozon refugee camp, 56–58, 61
GPFA Ebola Outreach Awareness Initiative (GEOAI), 174
Graff, Peter, 46, 120, 142, 158
Guinea: appeal for assistance, 147; case counts, 141; communication and social mobilization in, 125; economic effects in, 169–70; end of epidemic declaration, 178; first cases, 9; health care system challenges, 10; and IMS, 109; and Médecins Sans Frontières, 14, 116; and meeting of presidents, 43–44; testing in, 13; toll on, ix, xvii, 5, 9; travel restrictions and warnings, 43, 47–48; 2021 outbreak, 155; and World Bank support, 168–69. *See also* borders
Gurley, Emily, 191
Gwenigale, Walter T.: and IMS, 1, 76, 79–80, 103; and nomination of Tolbert Nyenswah as assistant minister, 90; and PREVAIL, 152; and task forces, 15–16, 193–94

Harris, James, 33, 34
Harris, Jugbeh, 34
hazard pay, 13, 136–37, 168, 169
health care system: collapse of, xi, 3, 5–6, 75–78, 157, 178–79; distrust of, x, 77, 179, 180; lack of treatment for other diseases, 167, 179; recovery and resilience building, xv–xvi, 3, 179–83. *See also* Ebola treatment units; laboratories; testing; treatment
health care workers: and community health workers, 18, 141, 159, 186; and COVID-19, 202; death benefits for, 137, 169; deaths of, 13, 77, 164; Ebola treatment unit for, 117–18; evacuations of Western, x–xi, 2, 42–43, 44–45, 48, 116, 140, 175; and hazard pay, 13, 136–37, 168, 169; infections of, 43, 48, 77, 117–18; international volunteers, 136, 144–45, 162, 163, 164–65; meeting with Sirleaf, 78–79; and refusal to treat, xi, 75, 77–78, 178–79; and refusal to work, xi, 3, 13; and

resiliency building, 180, 181; strikes by, 13, 78, 136, 168; training of, 141, 151, 164–65, 202
health centers, 93
Health Sector Coordination Committee, 180
Health Workers Association of Liberia, 168
helmet laws, 88
Henderson, Victor, 85, 88
Hill, Andrew, 149
Hill, Jah Lawrence, 38
HIV/AIDS, 87, 90, 129
hospitals: *vs.* health centers, 93; transmission in, 11–12, 43. *See also* Ebola treatment units

immunizations, 90
incident management system (IMS): appointment of Tolbert Nyenswah to, xiii, 1–2, 79–80, 91, 197; and case management, xiii, 103, 106, 108, 112, 115–19, 125; and CDC, 75–77, 91, 101, 102, 104, 109; communication and messaging, 106, 114–15, 123–30; and community engagement, xiv, 99, 103, 108, 113–15, 123–30; and contact tracing, xiii, 103, 105, 108, 111–15; county operations, 103, 105–7, 118; and COVID-19, 203–4; creation of, xiii, 75–77, 101–2, 194, 195; and dead body management, xiv, 103, 108, 109, 112, 116, 132–34; and decentralization, 105–7, 109; decision-making in, 101, 102, 107; development of concept, 103; and elections, 198; finances and accounting, 135; and laboratories, 103, 108, 112, 130–31; lessons learned, 194–98; and logistics, 103, 104, 112, 134–35; and media, 171–73; and nutritional support, 103, 118–19; and psychosocial support, xiv, 103, 106, 112, 131–32; and research, 152–53; and research credit, 196–97; and schools, 199; and self-reliance, 120; and social mobilization, xiv, 103, 106, 108, 112, 113–15, 123–30; structure of, xiii–xiv, 103–9, 112; and surveillance, xiii, 103, 108, 112, 119–23, 141; and testing, xiii–xiv, 103, 108, 130–31; and worker safety, 105, 106

incubation period, 8, 108, 111

infection prevention and control (IPC): and CDC, 151, 188; and COVID-19, 202; and Dead Body Management Team, 38; IMS focus on, 108, 125; initial lack of, 11–12, 13, 77; international support for, 141, 151, 157, 159, 162, 171; and nutritional support, 119; and recovery, 183, 185

Institute of Tropical Medicine Pedro Kouri, 164–65

Integrated Disease Surveillance and Response (IDSR), 183

International Association of National Public Health Institutes (IANPHI), 183, 185, 186

International Federation of Red Cross and Red Crescents, xv, 15, 132–33, 161, 167, 175

International Health Regulations (IHR), 6–7, 183

International Monetary Fund, 170

International Organization for Migration (IOM), 174

International Rescue Committee (IRC), 174

International Research & Exchanges Board (IREX), 129

international responses and support: and agendas, 196; and communication and social mobilization, 124, 127–30, 155, 169, 173–76; and contact tracing, 144, 145, 169, 174, 175; and declaration of emergency by WHO, xii–xiii, 4, 47, 48, 158; and Ebola treatment units, xiv, 12, 15, 115–16, 148–50, 155–58, 162–63, 165–66, 169, 175; and evacuation of Western personnel, x–xi, 2, 42–43, 44–45, 48, 116, 140, 175; fear of international transmission and foreign aid, x, 47–48, 140; and infection prevention and control, 141, 151, 157, 159, 162, 171; as initially slow, 14–15, 42–46, 116–17, 140, 195; and international volunteers, 136, 144–45, 162, 163, 164–65; and lack of experience with Ebola, 120, 139–40, 196; and leadership lessons, 195–98; and logistics, 134, 147, 149, 159, 161, 166, 170–71, 174; overview of, xiii, xiv–xv, 4; and PPE, 155–56, 159, 169; and psychosocial

support, 159, 176; and recovery stage, 178; and research papers, 196–97; and Sirleaf's request for help message, 3–4, 141–42, 166; and testing and laboratories, 130–31, 145, 161, 200; and transportation, 134, 159, 160, 163, 171. *See also* funding and aid

Investment Plan for Building a Resilient Health System, xv–xvi, 180–83

Island Clinic, 17–18, 143, 148

isolation: as basic to Ebola control, 108; and COVID-19 pandemic, 202; fear of, 4; first isolation units, 9; lack of isolation units, 12, 96; and monitoring, 113; and RITE, xv, 104, 118; in West Point and security issues, xi–xii, 92–101, 114. *See also* Ebola treatment units

Jackson, Samuel P., 22

Jacob Hughes Foundation, 102

Jallah, Dorbor, 134, 194

Johns Hopkins Bloomberg School of Public Health, 17, 89, 187

Johns Hopkins Center for Communication Programs, 175

Johns Hopkins Center for Health Security, 188

Johns Hopkins COVID-19 Contact Tracing Course, 190–91

Jones, Joel J., 84, 86

Kamara, Adulai, 172

Kamara, Shacki, 97

Karzon, Toagoe, 39

Kateh, Francis, 102, 118

Kennedy, Stephen B., 152

Kiboung, Richard Valery Mouzoko, 110

Kikeh, Annie, 70–72, 85, 88

Kikeh, Beatrice, 64, 66, 68–71, 72, 85

Kikeh, Dominic, 64, 66, 69–70, 73, 85

Kikeh, Josephine. *See* Nyenswah, Josephine

Kikeh, Patricia, 71

Kim, Jim Yong, 168–69

Ki-moon, Ban, 158

Kissi Camp, 39

Korha, Henry, 131

Koroma, Ernest Bai, 147, 169, 170

Korvayan, Mark Y., 38, 133

Kporkpoh, Francis, 177
Kru language, 64
Kulah, Arthur Flomo, 31
Kumeh, Humphrey C., 60–61, 63, 69
Kumeh, Munah, 60–61, 68

laboratories: and building resiliency, 180,
    181, 182, 183, 186, 201; and IMS, 103,
    108, 112, 130–31; international support
    for, 142, 161; National Reference
    Laboratory, 13, 130, 200, 201
Lagos Plan of Action for Economic
    Development of Africa, 24
Lane, H. Clifford, 152, 184, 186
Last Mile Health, 175
law, 86, 184
leadership: and COVID-19, 188–91, 202–4;
    and father's belief in Tolbert Nyenswah,
    x, 1, 26, 31–32, 80, 192; lessons learned,
    xvi, 194–204; of Ellen Johnson Sirleaf,
    189–90, 194–98; Ellen Johnson Sirleaf
    on Tolbert Nyenswah's, xvii–xviii
Liberia: civil wars, 10–11, 35, 49, 50–58, 60,
    83–84; coup (1980), 23; GDP, 10; health
    care system challenges, 10, 13; national
    anthem, 207; political history, 20–28;
    population distribution, 11
Liberia Crusaders for Peace, 175
Liberia Institute of Biomedical Research
    (LIBR), 13, 130, 131, 186
Liberia Medical and Dental Council
    (LMDC), 117, 168
Liberian National Coast Guard, xii, 98
Liberian Peace Council (LPC), 51–52
Liberian Red Cross, xv, 15, 175
Lift Liberia, Poverty Reduction Strategy, 181
literacy, 10, 124, 141
literacy, computer, 82
logistics: and border controls, 138; and
    IMS, 103, 104, 112, 134–35; international
    support for, 134, 147, 149, 159, 161, 166,
    170–71, 174; and recovery, 171. See also
    transportation
Louis Arthur Grimes School of Law, 86

Malac, Deborah, 47, 147, 148, 149, 165
malaria: and CDC, 87, 185; and medical
    volunteers, 164; messaging on, 129;

National Malaria Control Program, 84,
    86–87, 89, 90; symptoms, 9
Marathon, Monrovia, xvii, 205–6
Marburgvirus, 8
Massaquoi, Moses, 15, 117, 162, 174
Matthews, Gabriel Baccus, 25
Meal-A-Day School, 81
Médecins Sans Frontières (MSF): criticism
    by, 76; and Ebola treatment units, xiv,
    15, 115–16, 150, 155, 156–58; and EU aid,
    161; experience with Ebola, 139; job with,
    71; support overview, xiv, 45, 155–58; and
    testing, 200; warnings by, 14; and WHO,
    117
media, 18, 125, 129–30, 171–73
medical countermeasures, 151–52. *See also*
    treatment
Medical Emergency Relief International
    (MERCI), 175
Medical Teams International, 175
Medica Mondiale, 176
medications: and PREVAIL, 153; regula-
    tions, 181; and research, 2, 153; and
    treatment of Westerners, 44–45, 48
Mercy Corps, 127–29, 175
Merkel, Angela, 166
messaging. *See* communication and
    messaging
military and police: and cremation site
    security, 41–42; and West Point security
    issues, xi–xii, 96–99
Ministry of Finance and Development
    Planning (MOFDP), 83, 136
Ministry of Health and Social Welfare
    (MOHSW): career at, 80, 82–83, 84,
    86–91; Dead Body Management Team,
    x, 38–42; Disease Prevention Division,
    9, 17; finances and accounting, 102–3;
    fire at, 41; initial response, 6, 12–19, 37,
    193–94; Investment Plan for Building a
    Resilient Health System, xv–xvi, 180–83;
    and National Public Health Institute of
    Liberia, 185; and recovery, 179–83; and
    West Point isolation, xi–xii, 92–101, 114.
    See also incident management system
Ministry of Information, Cultural Affairs,
    and Tourism (MICAT), 171–72, 173
misdiagnoses, 6

misinformation, 18, 92–93, 123
missionaries, evacuation of, x–xi, 2, 44–45
Monrovia: Marathon, xvii, 205–6;
    population of, 11; post–civil war, 81;
    sanitation in, 11, 81
Monrovia Declaration, 24
Monrovia Medical Unit, 117, 148, 149
Moore, Gyude, 62
Moses, James Soka, 165–66
mosquito nets, 86, 129
motorcycles and safety, 88, 90–91
Mulbah, John, 117
Muyembe, Jean-Jacques, xvii, 145, 146, 204
Myers, Snoh, 62

Nabarro, David, 107, 115–16, 158
Nagbe, Thomas, 9, 107
National AIDS Control Program (NACP), 90
National Consultative Stakeholders, 180
National Council of Chiefs and Elders, 174
National Elections Commission (NEC), 198
National Health Policy and Plan, 180, 181
National Institute of Allergy and Infectious
    Diseases (NIAID), US, 154, 184
National Institutes of Health (NIH), US,
    48, 130, 150, 151–55, 184
National Malaria Control Program
    (NMCP), 84, 86–87, 89, 90
National Public Health Institute of Liberia
    (NPHIL), xix, xvi, 145, 183–86, 200, 201
National Reference Laboratory (NRL), 13,
    130, 200, 201
National Security Council (US), 147
National Tuberculosis Control Program
    (NTBCP), 87, 90
National Unification Policy, 21
Ndayimirije, Nestor, 16, 45, 46, 76, 91, 142,
    146
Neufville, A. Wa-Nyebo, 128–29
Ngafuan, Augustine Kpehe, 162
NGOs (nongovernmental organizations),
    support by, 104, 115, 173–76
Nicolo, Jorge Lefebre, 164
Nigeria: and Africa Centres for Disease
    Control and Prevention, 147; deaths in,
    142; and Sawyer case, 42–43; and second
    civil war in Liberia, 84; spread of Ebola
    from, 2, 143

nongovernmental organizations (NGOs),
    support by, 104, 115, 173–76
Nuclear Threat Initiative, 188
Nyenswah, Abraham, 55
Nyenswah, Agnes, 35, 50, 59
Nyenswah, Dehkontee, 85
Nyenswah, Josephine, 64–74, 83, 84–85, 91,
    187
Nyenswah, Martha, 27
Nyenswah, Moses, 27–28
Nyenswah, Nyennekon, 85
Nyenswah, Robert, 27, 81
Nyenswah, Ruth Tanneh Moses, 20, 27, 29,
    30, 71–72
Nyenswah, Sarah, 27
Nyenswah, Sharon, 50
Nyenswah, Suzanna, 27
Nyenswah, Swen, 55
Nyenswah, Tolbert, Jr., 89
Nyenswah, Tolbert Geewleh: appointment
    as deputy minister, 183; appointment as
    IMS manager, xiii, 1–2, 79–80, 91, 197;
    career, 17, 80–91, 183, 187–88; childhood,
    29–30, 32–36, 52–53; children of, 85, 89;
    education of, 17, 30, 32, 33, 60–63, 73–74,
    85–86, 88, 89; and grandparents, 28–29,
    52–53, 56; and marriage, 84–85; and
    name, 20, 21, 26; and Presidential Task
    Force on Ebola, 16–17, 76; and PREVAIL,
    186; threats to family, 187, 191
Nyenswah, Tolbert Geewleh, as refugee:
    and education, 60–63; and Gozon camp,
    56–59; and internal displacement of
    family, 50–55; return to Liberia, 73–74,
    80–81; Sirleaf on, ix–x; in Tabou, 60–73;
    and work, 51, 55, 57, 59–60
Nyenswah, William K. Moses: career,
    26–27, 31; and death of mother, 28–29;
    education of, 30; name, 30–31; and
    naming of Tolbert Nyenswah, 20, 21; and
    Tolbert Nyenswah, 21, 31; as refugee,
    50–54, 59, 61
Nyenswah, Wleh, 55
Nyenti, Mark E., 38

Obama, Barack, 147, 149
Office of Foreign Disaster Assistance
    (OFDA) of USAID, 104, 150–51

One Health approach, 140–41
"One Plan, One Strategy, One Response" slogan, xvi, 104–5, 196, 204
Operation United Assistance, 149
Organization of African Unity, 24. *See also* African Union
OSIWA (Open Society Initiative for West Africa), 176
Ouamouno, Emile, 6

Pajares, Miguel, xi, 45
palm oil trading, 55, 57, 59–60
Partnership for Research on Ebola Virus in Liberia (PREVAIL), 152–55, 186–87
Paul G. Allen Family Foundation, 128
Paye-layleh, Jonathan, 172
PCR (polymerase chain reaction) testing, 130, 131
Peace and Security Council of African Union, 144
Pence, Mike, 202
People's Redemption Council (PRC), 25–26
People's Republic of China. *See* China
personal protective equipment (PPE): challenges of, 115–16; and COVID-19, 202; and Dead Body Management Team, 39; and Ebola treatment units, 115–16, 155–56; and IMS, 105, 106; international support for, 155–56, 159, 169; lack of, 11, 78; transport of, 135
Peters, David, 187–88
Peters, Sarah, 52
phones: access to, 115, 121, 159, 174; feedback loop telephone system, 131–32
Piot, Peter, 145, 204
Population Services International (PSI), 129
Porte, Albert, 22
PPE. *See* personal protective equipment
pregnancy, refusal to treat, xi, 77–78, 178–79
Presidential Advisory Council on Ebola (PACE): and CDC, 147; and elections, 198; and health care workers' issues, 136; and IMS reporting, 104; and NGOs, 176; organizational chart, 112

Presidential Task Force on Ebola: criticism of, 76; establishment of, 15; fragmentation of, 17, 193–94; structure of, 16–17
President's Malaria Initiative (PMI), US, 87
PREVAIL (Partnership for Research on Ebola Virus in Liberia), 152–55, 186–87
Progressive Alliance of Liberia (PAL), 25
psychosocial support: and IMS, xiv, 103, 106, 112, 131–32; international support for, 159, 176

quarantines: and Dolo's Town, 92, 95; in Nigeria, 42; and West Point and security issues, xi–xii, 92–101, 114. *See also* Ebola treatment units; isolation
Quick, Jonathan D., 189–90

Railey, Kent, 33, 34
rapid isolation and treatment of Ebola (RITE), xv, 104, 118
recovery and resilience building, xv–xvi, 3, 171, 179–83, 205–6
Red Cross, xv, 15, 132–33, 161, 167, 175
Redemption Hospital, 11–12
refugee, Tolbert Nyenswah as. *See* Nyenswah, Tolbert Geewleh, as refugee
religious groups: and burials, 133; and community engagement, 126–27, 199–200; and COVID-19, 126; and Presidential Task Force on Ebola, 16
research: as limited, 7–8; and PREVAIL, 152–55, 186–87; research papers and credit, 196–97
resilience: building, xv–xvi, 3, 179–83; defined, 191; importance of, 191; investment plan for, xv–xvi, 180–83
Response Management Team of USAID, 150–51
Rice Riots, 22–23, 25
RITE (rapid isolation and treatment of Ebola), xv, 104, 118
Rosling, Hans, 120–23
Rouse, Edward N., 102
Russ, Cathy, 33–34
Russ, Florence, 33–34, 36
Russ, Hamilton C., III, 32
Russ, Nellie, 32–35
RVSV-ZEBOV vaccine, 153, 186

Samaritan's Purse, 12, 16, 44, 116, 175–76
sanitation: and building resiliency, 180, 181; international support for, 159, 173; in Monrovia, 11, 81; as refugee, 53, 54, 57; and transmission, 41
SARS, 185
Save the Children, 176
Sawyer, Patrick, x, 42–43, 47
Saye, Arthur A. D., 82–83
schools, 6, 15, 47, 50, 170, 198–99
scientists. *See* African scientists
seaports, 138
Search for Common Ground (SFCG) Liberia, 176
secret burials, x, 38, 42
security: and burial sites, 39–40; and cremation, 41–42; and West Point isolation, xi–xii, 92–101
self-reliance, 24, 120, 197
Serving in Mission (SIM), 12
Severe Infection Temporary Treatment Unit (SITTU), 166–67
sexual transmission, 165
Sharfstein, Joshua, 191
Sierra Leone: appeal for assistance, 147; case counts, 141; civil war (1991–2002), 84; communication and social mobilization in, 125; economic effects of epidemic, 169–70; end of epidemic declaration, 178; and EU aid, 161; first cases, 9; health care system challenges, 10; and IMS, 109; and Médecins Sans Frontières, 116; and meeting of presidents, 43–44; persistence of outbreaks in, 178; toll on, ix, xvii, 5, 9; travel restrictions and warnings, 43, 47–48; and World Bank support, 168–69. *See also* borders
Sirleaf, Ellen Johnson: and Africa Centres for Disease Control and Prevention, 145, 147; appeal for international help, 3–4, 141–42, 166; appeal to US, 147; appointment of Tolbert Nyenswah to IMS, xiii, 1, 79, 197; and Brussels Airlines, 138; and celebration of end of epidemic, 177; commencement speech, 193; cremation mandate, x, 41–42, 133; criticism of, 14, 123, 189; curfew declaration, xi, xii, 47, 98; on economic recovery, 170; foreword by, ix–xviii; and IMS creation, xiii–xiv, 194, 195; and IMS reporting, 103, 104; leadership of, 189–90, 194–98; on leadership of Tolbert Nyenswah, xvii–xviii; and meeting of presidents, 43–44; meeting with health care workers, 78–79; and National Public Health Institute of Liberia, xvi, 184, 186; and Operation United Assistance meeting, 149; Presidential Task Force on Ebola creation, 15; on resilience building, xv–xvi; state of emergency declaration, xi, xii, 47, 189–90; and treatment of Western personnel, 44; on volunteers from other African countries, 145; and West Point quarantine, xi–xii, 94–95, 98
SITTU (Severe Infection Temporary Treatment Unit), 166–67
Slewion, Harrison, 81–82
soccer, 63–64
social mobilization: and contact tracing, 113–15; and COVID-19 pandemic, 202, 203; defined, 199; field reports, 127; importance of, 199–200, 203; and IMS, xiv, 103, 106, 108, 112, 113–15, 123–30; international support for, 155, 169, 173–76; and malaria, 87; and media, 125, 129–30, 171–73; and Presidential Task Force on Ebola, 18, 76; and vaccine trials, 153
social services, closing of, 198–99
Spain, evacuations by, xi, 45, 140
Star of the Sea health center, 93
state of emergency declaration, xi, xii, 47, 189–90
state-owned enterprises, 184
stigma, 4, 121, 125, 127
Stone, Mardia, xix, 196
strikes, 13, 78, 136, 168
Sudan ebolavirus, 8
Sumo, John, 18, 124
surveillance: and building resiliency, 180, 181, 182, 183; course at Emory University, 88; and data management, 13; and Global Health Security Agenda, 141; and IMS, xiii, 103, 108, 112, 119–23, 141
survivors: acceptance of, 129; and antibodies, 9; criteria for release, 156, 157;

discharge celebrations, 162–63; Ebola Survivor's Clinic, 165; follow-up treatment for, 156–57; and long-term health effects, 153; stigma of, 125, 127; testimonies by, 130

Tabou: Tolbert Nyenswah as refugee in, 60–73; refugee camp, 58
Taylor, Charles, 31, 50, 73, 84
teaching. *See* tutoring by Tolbert Nyenswah
testing: and building resiliency, xv–xvi, 180, 181, 182, 183, 186; capacity, 13, 200; and COVID-19, 200, 202; and IMS, xiii–xiv, 103, 108, 130–31; international support for, 130–31, 161, 200; negative tests, 156; and transportation, 130, 131, 135, 200
Tetteh, Hanna Serwaa, 177–78
Toe, Albert, 25
Togba, Harrison, 64–69, 71
toilets. *See* sanitation
Tolbert, Stephen, Sr., 22
Tolbert, William R., Jr., 20, 21–25, 31
Tony Blair Africa Governance Initiative / Tony Blair Institute for Global Change, 176
touching and transmission, x, 18–19, 129
traditional practices. *See* funeral and burial practices
transmission: across borders, 9–10, 15; fear of international transmission and foreign aid, x, 47–48, 140; and funeral and burial practices, x, 7, 11, 37–38, 132, 199–200; in hospitals, 11–12, 43; and lag in testing, 13; and sanitation, 41; and secret burials, x, 38, 42; sexual, 165; and touching, x, 18–19, 129; vectors of, 7
transportation: airline stoppages, 3, 43, 138; and border controls, 138; and burial teams, 39, 133; and IMS logistical services, 134; international support for, 134, 159, 160, 163, 171; and motorcycle safety, 88, 90–91; and screenings, 138, 203; and testing, 130, 131, 135, 200; as transmission vector, 7
travel restrictions and warnings, 3, 43, 47–48, 138, 143

treatment: and ASEOWA, 145; follow-up treatment, 156–57; as limited, 7–8; and National Institutes of Health (US), 48, 151–55; and PREVAIL, 152–55; refusal to treat, xi, 75, 77–78, 178–79; and RITE, xv, 104, 118; supportive, 8, 9, 117; of Western personnel, x–xi, 2, 44–45, 48, 117–18. *See also* Ebola treatment units; medications; vaccines
Trump, Donald J., 188, 203
tuberculosis, 87, 90
Tubman, William V. S., 20–21, 24
tutoring by Tolbert Nyenswah, 65–66, 71, 81, 83
Tweh, Stephen T., 82
Tyler, Alex, 16, 177

Uganda, outbreaks in, 13
UNICEF (United Nations International Children's Emergency Fund), 129–30, 159–60
United Nations: foreign aid estimates, 195; and IMS, 107; initial response, 46; and refugees, 56, 58–59, 62, 63, 73–74; response overview, xv, 158–59; and second civil war in Liberia, 84
United Nations Development Programme (UNDP), 113, 114, 136, 179
United Nations High Commission on Refugees (UNHCR), 56, 58–59, 62, 63, 73–74
United Nations International Children's Emergency Fund (UNICEF), 129–30, 159–60
United Nations Mission for Ebola Emergency Response (UNMEER), 107, 120, 158–59
United Nations Office of Project Services (UNOPS), 160
United Nations Population Fund (UNFPA), 77–78
United Nations Programme on HIV/AIDS (UNAIDS), 87
United States: and China aid, 161–62; and COVID-19, 188–91, 198, 202–4; evacuations by, x–xi, 2, 44–45, 140; funding by, 151, 186; and Global Health Security Agenda, 140; infections in, 48, 203; initial response, 14–15; Liberia

United States (*cont.*)
  policy and involvement, 23–24, 25; and Deborah Malac, 47, 147, 148; and Monrovia Medical Unit, 117, 148, 149; move to by Tolbert Nyenswah, 187; and National Public Health Institute of Liberia, 186; overview of support from, xv, 147–55, 159. *See also specific agencies*
Universal Declaration of Human Rights (UDHR), 87–88
University of Liberia, 83, 86
USAID (US Agency for International Development): and community engagement, 127–29; Disaster Assistance Response Team, 104, 147, 149–51, 160; and IMS, 104, 127–29; initial response, 14–15, 45; and malaria, 87; Office of Foreign Disaster Assistance, 104, 150–51; support overview, xv, 147, 149–51, 160
US Army Corps of Engineers, 150
US Army Medical Research Institute of Infectious Diseases, 130
US Department of Defense, xv, 117, 149–50
US Department of Health and Human Services, 152–55, 187
US Public Health Service, 117, 150

vaccines: for Ebola, 2, 7, 152–55, 186–87; vaccination rates, 179
van der Groen, Guido, 204
viral hemorrhagic fever. *See* Ebola virus disease

Wapoe, Jacob, 39
water: and Ebola treatment units, 149, 150; lack of as challenge, 78, 81; and NGOs, 173; and quarantines, 95
Welthungerhilfe, 176
Wesseh, C. Stanford, 113
West African Health Organization (WAHO), 180
Western personnel: evacuation of, x–xi, 2, 42–43, 44–45, 48, 116, 140, 175; treatment of, x–xi, 44–45, 48, 117–18

West Point slum and security issues, xi–xii, 92–101, 114
WHO (World Health Organization): case estimates, 142; and community engagement, 144; and contact tracing, 144; criticism of, 139; and Dead Body Management Team, 38; declaration of end of epidemic, 141, 177–78, 182; declaration of public health emergency, 4, 47, 48, 158, xii–xiii; and DRC, 110; and EU aid, 161; experience with Ebola, 139; and Guinea 2021 outbreak, 155; and IMS, 91, 104, 107, 142; initial response, 14–15, 37, 45, 142; International Health Regulations, 6–7, 183; leadership changes in region, 45, 46, 142; and Médecins Sans Frontières, 117; and meeting of presidents, 43–44; and National Public Health Institute of Liberia, 184, 186; and Presidential Task Force on Ebola, 16; and recovery, 178, 179, 180, 181–82; reporting obligations, 6–7; response overview, xiv, 142–43; and transportation, 160; and treatment, 143–44, 150, 155, 165
Williams, Darryl, 149
Williams, Desmond, 178, 184
Woods, Kofi, 100
worker safety and IMS, 105, 106. *See also* personal protective equipment
World Bank, xv, 24, 136, 167–70, 180
World Food Programme, 134, 170–71
World Health Organization. *See* WHO
Writebol, Nancy, x–xi, 44–45

Yett, Sheldon, 159–60
Yue, Zhang, 162
Yungui, Wang, 162

Zagursky, Rony, 194
Zaire ebolavirus, 8
Zarif, Farid, 186
Zinner, Lauren, 174
ZMapp, 44, 153

Milton Keynes UK
Ingram Content Group UK Ltd.
UKHW011052270923
429432UK00001B/1